STOP AGING NOW!

NUMBER ONE WITH DOCTORS
AND WINNER OF THE 1995 EXCELLENCE IN JOURNALISM AWARD
FROM THE AMERICAN AGING ASSOCIATION

"Provocative, lively, well-written . . . *Stop Aging Now!* will add to the public's education about nutrition, disease, and aging."—Robert Butler, M.D., chairman of the department of geriatrics, Mount Sinai School of Medicine

"There is little doubt that the aging process can be slowed or even reversed, Ms. Carper's provocative book will undoubtedly spark physicians and scientists to accelerate much-needed aging research."—Stephen DeFelice, M.D., chairman of the Foundation for Innovation in Medicine

"A wonderful book, scientifically accurate—a major resource for the public and professionals who are interested in factors contributing to aging and [how to] decrease the risk and stay healthy."—John Weisburger, Ph.D., cancer researcher, director emeritus, the American Health Foundation

"Jean Carper is one of the most reliable authorities on ways of improving health by natural means. I recommend her books to my patients and students."—Andrew T. Weil, M.D., University of Arizona School of Medicine, author of *Spontaneous Healing*

"I liked *Stop Aging Now!* so much I also bought copies for my mother and mother-in-law."—Michael Meguid, M.D., professor of surgery and neuroscience, State University of New York Health Science Center, Syracuse, and editor-in-chief of *Nutrition, the International Journal of Applied and Basic Nutritional Sciences*

"So far I have bought 215 copies of *Stop Aging Now!* for patients and friends. It's the best book I've ever seen on diet, health, and longevity."—Daniel N. Tucker, M.D., allergist and immunologist, Good Samaritan Hospital, West Palm Beach, Florida

ALSO BY JEAN CARPER

Food—Your Miracle Medicine
The Food Pharmacy
The Food Pharmacy Guide to Good Eating

STOP AGING NOW!

THE ULTIMATE PLAN FOR STAYING YOUNG AND REVERSING THE AGING PROCESS

Jean Carper

HarperPerennial
A Division of HarperCollins*Publishers*

HarperCollins books may be purchased for educational, business, or sales promotional use. For information, please write: Special Markets Department, HarperCollins Publishers, Inc., 10 East 53rd Street, New York, NY 10022.

First HarperPerennial edition published 1996.

Designed by Laura Lindgren

The Library of Congress has catalogued the hardcover edition as follows:

Carper, Jean
　　Stop aging now! : the ultimate plan for staying young and
　reversing the aging process / Jean Carper.
　　　　p.　cm.
　　Includes bibliographical references and index.
　　ISBN 0-06-018355-1
　　1. Longevity.　2. Aging.　3. Health.　I. Title.
　RA776.75.C37　　1996
　612.6'8—dc20　　　　　　　　　　　　　　　　95-193611

ISBN 0-06-098500-3 (pbk.)

98 99 ❖/RRD 10 9

To Joan, Judy, Larry, Bob, Natella, Thea

CONTENTS

THE STUFF THAT ROBS YOU OF YOUR YOUTH

THE DANGER SIGNS OF NEEDLESS AGING—ANTIDOTES AND REMEDIES

ACKNOWLEDGMENTS

The author of this book is a conduit of ideas, representing a synthesis of the current thinking of many scientists. For nearly two decades I have been privileged as a medical journalist to be able to tap into the flow of new theories and research about the importance of antioxidants, free radicals, and other substances in food; about health supplements; and now about aging, the most monumental human health concern of all. The scientists, numbering in the thousands, with whom I have had contact during that time have added to the range of ideas that have culminated in this book.

In particular I want to mention some who have been most influential in pioneering and shaping the ideas presented in *Stop Aging Now!* Some of the scientists were new to me when I started this book; some have been in my Rolodex for years.

When I first started researching this book, the name that popped up everywhere in writings on free radicals and aging was Denham Harman, M.D., now acknowledged as the man who, forty years ago, first thought of the free radical theory of aging. He and his wife, Helen, have been taking supplements almost since that time and are testaments to the validity of Dr. Harman's pioneering ideas and research. To Dr. Harman, both I and the world owe a very big thanks for discovering and telling us how we can save ourselves from some of the sufferings of aging.

Others who have added greatly to this book and scientific knowledge about aging and age-related diseases, although they are not always specifically credited in the text, are: Dr. John Weisburger, who first at the National Cancer Institute and now at American Health Foundation has continued to enlighten me about the intricacies of antioxidants and carcinogens. Dr. Mary Enig, formerly a scientist at the University of Maryland, who recognized the dangers of polyunsaturated fats and trans fatty acids as far back as 1980, virtually before anyone else. Dr. Dean Jones, Emory University researcher on glutathione, who has patiently explained to me the many attributes of this powerful antioxidant. Dr. William Lands, now at the National Institutes of Health, my mentor on the chemistry and health aspects of fatty acids—namely the omega-3s and omega-6s. And what would life be without the many scientists from Harvard's School of Public Health and the U.S. Department of Agriculture's Human Nutrition Research Center on Aging at Tufts University. They have done much pioneering work in the area of nutrients, health, and aging. In particular, Dr. Charles Hennekens and Dr. Walter Willett at Harvard; and at Tufts Drs. Simin and Moshen Meydani and Dr. Jeffrey Blumberg. Also among the prominent pioneers in free radicals, antioxidants, aging and age-related diseases are Dr. Bruce Ames and Dr. Gladys Block at the University of California, Berkeley, and Dr. Roy Walford at UCLA, whose work and public pronouncements have done much to further the understanding of aging and age-related diseases.

My gratitude also to the scientists who reviewed portions of this book before publication.

Thanks to my publisher, Gladys Justin Carr, whose vision made this book possible, and to my agent, Raphael Sagalyn, who is surely the best, most caring, meticulous, and enthusiastic agent an author can want. Again, for helping me fashion the organization and content of the book during the writing of the manuscript, my gratitude to my longtime best editor and friend, Thea Flaum.

INTRODUCTION

Youth Potions Are Here Now—
and They're Yours for the Taking

▲   ▲   ▲   ▲   ▲   ▲   ▲

> Aging—the detrimental changes that occur as you get older—is actually in large part a monumental, progressive deficiency disease. It begins in adulthood, picks up in middle age and takes a giant leap after age fifty. You can prevent and correct it to an amazing extent, preserving and reclaiming your youth and vigor and stretching your life span.

If there was a magic potion to preserve youth, who wouldn't take it? Yet the prospect of youth potions is no longer remote. In fact, such awesome agents are here now. The staggering truth is that scientists have already identified scores of substances that strike at the very heart of aging by slowing down and even reversing the deterioration that we now view as normal aging. And, although you may not realize it, you have wide access to virtually all these youth potions.

The incredible powers of these antiaging potions are being uncovered every day in prestigious laboratories worldwide—and they are easily obtainable and remarkably safe. They are in your food, in your vitamin bottle, and in your health food store. And they cost very little, especially when compared to the monumental cost of *not* taking them.

Unimaginable as it may seem, it is within your control to maintain or recapture many of the faculties and state of well-being that traditionally slip away with age. For the first time in history, scientists are increasingly focusing not just on combating individual diseases but on the entire process of aging and what it really is—an instant by instant destruction of weakened, undefended cells that on a massive scale leads to a regrettable and frightening global degeneration of body and mind.

But such aging, science now suspects, is not inevitable, or even natural. It is, in fact, an unnatural human condition that to a startling degree is preventable and treatable.

Many prominent investigators now view aging not as an inevitable consequence of time, but as a disease itself—the ultimate conglomerate disease caused by a lifetime of environmental assaults to cells, leading to a slow degeneration of the body and culminating in multiple breakdowns of bodily functions (what we now call chronic diseases). Like all disease processes, aging can be slowed down and sometimes even reversed. There is mounting evidence that you can interfere at all ages with this deterioration. It is never too early or too late to try to interrupt this process.

THE ANTIAGING FRONTIER

The implications of the exploding inquiries into aging causes and cures are staggering and not yet generally appreciated. Scientists can now proclaim truthfully that, after centuries of humankind's search for the elusive fountain of youth, they have located part of it deep within the genetic makeup of cells. There in the DNA, many think, resides a primary cause of aging and a way to slow it down. The discovery could be historic in controlling human destiny and longevity.

For example, the "antioxidant vitamins" you hear so much about as useful in warding off cancer, heart disease, arthritis and neurological diseases all have a single underlying mechanism that works by stifling damage-induced aging within cells. In short, the way foods and herbs often fight cancer and other chronic diseases is by fighting aging. Thus, most antidisease diet-connected research ultimately focuses on a single outcome: to forestall the degeneration we call aging. Scientists, by reaching deep into the molecular biology of cells, are discovering the body's aging controls and ways to turn down the aging process, using, of all things, nature's own agents that are in vast supply in food and plants.

In the September 1993 issue of the *Proceedings of the National Academy of Sciences*, a leading pioneer in the subject, Dr. Bruce N. Ames of the University of California, Berkeley, laid out the theory in a review called "Oxidants, Antioxidants and the Degenerative Diseases of Aging." His point: that oxidative damage to the cells' genetic DNA accumulates with age and is a major contributor to aging and to the degenerative diseases of aging, including cancer, cardiovascular disease, immune-system decline and brain and nervous system dysfunction, such as Parkinson's disease, Lou Gehrig's disease, and cerebral vascular changes that we know as "senility." The astonishing news, he says, is that these DNA mutations that accumulate with age can be partially blocked by eating the right antioxidants found in foods, thus slowing down the process of deterioration in numerous ways.

Additionally, academic scientists, some at federal government-supported aging research centers such as that at

Tufts University, have identified many age-related bodily changes that predict disease. With age, your body undergoes various biochemical changes that have been mistakenly accepted as the inevitable consequences of aging when instead they are signs of deterioration and disease that can be dramatically reversed, sometimes by a modest dose of common nutrients.

For example, as you age, you are apt to produce more of a substance in the blood called homocysteine, which is inclined to make blood clot more easily, leading to heart attacks. In fact, many heart attack patients have normal cholesterol but high levels of homocysteine. Amazingly, folic acid, rich in foods like spinach, and doses of B6 quickly reduce homocysteine, partially erasing the "aging factor" and thus, logically, the threat of heart disease.

It's also well known that immune functioning breaks down as we get older and is thought to be a prime reason for more infections, as well as cancer, in the elderly. However, a recent groundbreaking study by leading immunologist Ranjit K. Chandra at Memorial University of Newfoundland found that a supplement of modest doses of eighteen common vitamins and minerals dramatically boosted immune functioning and cut infectious illnesses in half among a group of elderly people. His finding is heralded as a major breakthrough by the mainstream medical community.

Similarly, during middle age, the thymus gland, a major player in immune functioning, begins to shrink dramatically, coinciding with a decline in production of thymulin, a hormone that creates disease-fighting T-cells. Yet several studies find that only 30 daily milligrams of zinc rejuvenated the functioning of the thymus gland in people over age sixty-five, restoring their output of thymulin and T-cell production to equal that of people twenty years younger.

Even more astounding is the potential reversal of age-related brain dysfunction. Losing mental faculties as we age is tragic and common. However, new research indicates that memory loss, lack of concentration and confusion can often be traced to deficiencies in vitamins, mainly the B vitamins, such as vitamin B12, B6 and folic acid. Several studies have found that as many as 20 to 30 percent of those diagnosed with Alzheimer's disease and other types of dementia actually had a vitamin B12 deficiency. They recovered their mental capacities when given the vitamin. Many experts recommend that everyone suspected of failing mental functions be tested for vitamin B deficiencies. With age, many stop producing a stomach enzyme required to absorb vitamin B12 in food and thus need supplements. Much mental deterioration associated with aging can be prevented or reversed by vitamins, declares Dr. Irwin H. Rosenberg of the U.S. Department of Agriculture's Human Nutrition Research Center on Aging at Tufts University.

Moreover, physicians in Europe have documented spectacular rejuvenation in memory and general mental competence in older people by using the leaf of a ginkgo tree to stimulate blood circulation in the brain.

In this book you will discover every scientifically valid dietary substance—and the dose—to forestall aging throughout your life.

All this does not mean you will live forever or achieve immortality. Most scientists are convinced that nature has built in a maximum life span for all mammals, including humans, past which there is no trespassing. (One hundred and twenty years, many think, is our ultimate boundary.) But you can strive for the most desired state—to die young as late as possible—to avoid what Charles de Gaulle called "the shipwreck of old age." Or as George Burns said: "You can't help getting older, but you don't have to get old." We no longer need consider Shakespeare's seventh age—sans teeth, sans hair, sans everything—as the inevitable penalty of a long life.

THE ANTIAGING REVOLUTION IS HERE NOW

By taking action to slow down your own aging, you are part of a marvelous revolution in medicine that emphasizes prevention instead of treatment. The irreversible reality is that we are living longer, and how we handle it makes a monumental difference to all of us. We can view aging as humankind's inevitable destiny and idly sit by as our bodies disintegrate. Or we can take action to hang on to and replenish our biochemical vitality that is slipping away. If you require more antioxidants and other substances to restock dwindling supplies in the face of aging's increased needs, why not take them now?

It's true that some advise waiting. They argue it's too soon to explore these newly discovered fountains of youth because science hasn't fully established how well they work. Some scientists feel they cannot risk their reputations by recommending antiaging agents to the entire public until every last scientific *i* has been dotted and every *t* crossed—until these substances are extensively tested the same way as potent pharmaceutical drugs—with so-called human randomized double-blind trials. That could take ten to twenty years and probably will never be done. Nevertheless, in the meantime, many scientists are taking megadoses of vitamins and other antiaging potions to minimize their own aging. On the other side, outspoken scientists such as Dr. Gladys Block, noted researcher at the University of California, think such clinical trials, used to test drugs, are irrelevant to evaluating preventive antioxidant vitamins and will never reveal the whole truth. Dr. Jeffrey Blumberg of Tufts says generations could pass before answers emerge from such trials.

Of utmost importance is whether there could be a danger to taking supplements. Most scientists see none. Many agree with Harvard's Dr. Walter Willett, who says it's foolish to wait when the stakes are so high and the risk so low. "I think it's perfectly rational to take supplements now because there's a good chance they will help and there seems to be no danger."

"The side effects [of taking megadoses of antioxidant vitamins] are zip. It's kind of a gamble where the downside is absolutely nothing," argues Steven Harris, M.D., associate research pathologist at UCLA, who says he takes vitamins E and C and "just enough beta carotene to turn the soles of my feet yellow."

The price of delay could be tragic. Consider scurvy, for example, one of the deadliest scourges of the Middle Ages. Scientists suspected for nearly two centuries that fruits rich in vitamin C prevented scurvy. In fact, it was proved beyond a doubt in the mid seventeen hundreds. Even then, it was another half century before the British government mandated that sailors at sea be given limes or lemons. In that interim, more than two hundred thousand British sailors died of scurvy.

Some think we are in a similar scientific waiting game over aging antidotes and remedies. If so, how long is too long to wait before taking action? Only you can decide for yourself.

Some scientists have adopted a "wait and see" attitude. Of course, if they wait too long, they won't see.

—Dr. Roy Walford, professor of pathology, University of California at Los Angeles Medical School

We're in a war. It's life against death, and we're all in the killing zone of the aging process. To do nothing is to be wiped out. —Dr. Ward Dean, clinical gerontologist in Florida, as quoted in *Life* magazine, October 1992

Americans are dying prematurely of heart disease and cancer. Are we so uncertain that we want to discourage supplements? Generations can pass before the answers are complete. —Dr. Jeffrey Blumberg, Tufts University, 1994

Cracking the Mystery
of Why We Age
and How We Can Stop It

If you know how free radicals are born and how to partially tame them, you understand the rules of the aging game and the simple moves you can make to help save yourself from premature and devastating aging.

Y ou age, as does every living creature. It is part of the cosmic plan. Aging is universal, as is death. But how rapidly you age is not. Nor is your own individual life span. Both the rate at which you age and your time on earth are under more control than you may dream—and than scientists envisioned until recently.

Exploding research into aging and related diseases is suddenly producing some awesome prospects. Recent discoveries are enough to take scientists' breath away—and ours—as they enter territory never before explored, witnessing at ever closer range the ultimate biological mysteries of life and death. These new investigations, for the first time in human history, promise ways to expand our mortality and avoid the curse of old age, allowing us to live at our fullest capacity until the end of our lives.

Free Radicals Cause Aging

Not surprisingly, the secrets of aging lie deep in the molecular biology of individual cells. There are admittedly several theories of aging, but one has emerged as the most compelling and best supported by impressive new evidence. This does not mean the theory necessarily accounts for all aging changes, but many authorities believe it explains a major part. It is called the free radical theory of aging, and it goes this way: Aging occurs when cells are permanently damaged by continual attacks from chemical particles called free radicals. Simply, the cellular damage accumulates over the years, until the totality of destruction reaches the point of no return—diseases clustered at the end of life and eventually death. This, then—the perpetual but futile struggle of individual cells to stay alive and function normally, in the face of chemical disintegration—is the genesis of aging and all its consequences.

THE PHENOMENAL FACTS

- ▲ The knowledge is here now! You can slow down the aging process and its consequences to some extent—no matter how old or how young you are.
- ▲ Think of aging and the diseases that tag after it as an unrecognized, untreated "deficiency disease" of incredible proportions. Then treat it.
- ▲ The unrecognized truth is that so many aging changes are needless and reversible!
- ▲ We think of a pathogen as a bacteria or virus that destroys our health. But the greatest pathogen of all is *time*.

This monumental revelation came to pioneering researcher Denham Harman, M.D., Ph.D., emeritus professor of medicine at the University of Nebraska College of Medicine, in a flash of insight in 1954. But, like most bold ideas, it was largely ignored until, after numerous groundbreaking experiments by Dr. Harman, a splurge of new research starting in the late sixties began to overwhelmingly validate it. Now it is heralded as a breakthrough theory in the study of aging. The idea fuels billions of dollars of research not only into aging per se, but into the diseases of aging, such as cancer and heart disease, all of which appear to owe their genesis to one identical source—free radicals.

Indeed, the free radical theory of aging is so big it encompasses virtually every disease you can think of that comes with increasing age. That, then, makes aging the primary and only disease most of us ever have to worry about. As Dr. Harman notes, we have pressed the life span about as far as it will go without attacking aging at its origin. We are at the point, he says, where "the major risk of death for anyone over about age twenty-eight in the U.S. is aging!"

In Dr. Harman's view, degenerative diseases such as cancer, heart disease, arthritis, Lou Gehrig's disease and Alzheimer's are not separate and distinguishable entities. They are merely different forms of expression, influenced by genetics and environment, of the free radical aging process that has caught up with us. Indeed, an estimated 80 to 90 percent of all degenerative diseases involve free radical activity, say some experts. Viewing them separately is like taking an aspirin to relieve the fever of an infection instead of an antibiotic to kill the bacteria. It misses the point. In short, virtually all our maladies are actually "accelerated aging." Slow down the aging and you eliminate or postpone the problems.

The Danger Is in the Air

Oxygen is what it is all about. Ironically, the stuff that gives us life eventually snuffs it out. The ultimate life force lies in tiny cellular factories of energy, called mitochondria, that burn nearly all the oxygen we breathe in. But breathing has a price. The combustion of oxygen that keeps us alive and active spews off by-products called oxygen free radicals. They have Dr. Jekyll and Mr. Hyde characteristics. On the one hand, they help guarantee our survival. For example, when the body mobilizes to fight off infectious agents, it generates a burst of free radicals to destroy the invaders very efficiently. On the other hand, free radicals, including the pervasive superoxides created by respiration, careen out of control through the body, attacking cells, turning their fats rancid, rusting their proteins, piercing their membranes and corrupting their genetic code until the cells become dysfunctional and sometimes give up and die. These fierce radicals, built into life as both protectors and avengers, are the potent agents of aging.

Additionally, we hasten our demise by taking in free radicals that originate outside our bodies. Smoking fills the body with free radicals. So do environmental pollutants. So does being in the sunlight and being exposed to radiation. In short, we are bombarded from within and without throughout life with these simultaneously life-preserving and life-erasing free radicals. We could not survive without them, but when they run amok in large forces, they make us old before our time and kill us sooner than later.

Chemically, free radicals are simply molecules that are missing an electron and are desperately trying to snatch one from any other molecule. In so doing, they become

ANTIAGING SECRETS OF THE EXPERTS

Denham Harman, M.D.: The First Pioneer
Emeritus Professor of Medicine
University of Nebraska College of Medicine

Dr. Harman was the first to propose the free radical theory of aging in 1954. Few paid any attention for decades. But he kept up his crusade, doing numerous studies on animals at the University of Nebraska where, now at age seventy-eight, he is emeritus professor of medicine.

Here's what Dr. Harman takes every day to postpone aging:

▲ Vitamin E—150 to 300 international units (IU).
▲ Vitamin C—2,000 milligrams, taken in 500-milligram doses four times a day.
▲ Beta carotene—25,000 IU (15 milligrams) every other day.
▲ Coenzyme Q-10—30 milligrams, taken in 10-milligram doses three times a day.
▲ Selenium—100 micrograms, taken in 50-microgram doses twice a day.
▲ Zinc—30 milligrams every other day.
▲ Magnesium—250 milligrams.
▲ A low-dose multiple-vitamin tablet *without iron.*

molecular terrorists. They can be neutralized by antioxidants, compounds that give up one of their electrons, thus returning the free radicals to normal and stopping their cellular mayhem.

THE ANTIOXIDANT ANSWER

Fortunately, the body does not easily knuckle under to these barrages of free radical assaults. It calls forth an arsenal of defenses, made up of enzymes and other chemicals called antioxidants. If the free radicals are the thugs of the body, the antioxidants are the police force. They are chemically designed to defuse the destructive free radicals. They do this by stopping their formation, snuffing them out and repairing their damage, which is ubiquitous and formidable. For example, about a trillion molecules of oxygen go through each cell every day, inflicting about one hundred thousand free radical hits or wounds on your cells' genes or DNA, estimates geneticist Bruce Ames of the University of California at Berkeley. The good news is patrolling antioxidant enzymes rush to snip out and repair the genes, erasing from 99 to 99.9 percent of the damage, Ames has shown. The bad news is, that still leaves one thousand new wounds every day that go unrepaired, and this damage accumulates relentlessly. "So by the time you're old, we find a few million oxygen lesions [wounds] per cell," says Ames. It is this accumulation of cellular damage or rubbish from incomplete repair that fuels the aging process, pushing up your odds of disease and death.

It's been estimated that by age fifty, about 30 percent of your cellular protein has been turned into rusty junk by free radical attacks. Particularly vulnerable also are fatty molecules, which are abundant in the delicate structural membranes of the cells and in the blood. Free radical attacks oxidize such fat, leaving it spoiled, just as butter out of the refrigerator becomes rancid. In a sense, it has been said that as we age, we chemically resemble a piece of meat that has been left too long in the open air and sun.

Through free radical reactions in our body, it's as though we're being irradiated at low levels all the time. They grind us down. —Lester Packer, biochemist at University of California at Berkeley, who has been studying free radicals since the 1970s

WHY WE CAN'T LIVE FOREVER

We can never escape aging because nature's plan builds it into our genes, some say, because nature cares little about us after forty or fifty, when we have performed our duties of reproduction, providing fresh gene pools for evolution. It becomes more difficult with time to fend off the free radicals that are taking away our youth.

In the natural, universal order of things, as we get older, two critical things happen biologically to hasten aging. The rate of increase of cell-damaging free radical reactions accelerates dramatically. Even worse news, your inborn abilities to defuse and repair the damage from the free radicals—your detoxification systems—lose steam also as you age. This means that the older you get, the more damage accumulates in your cells and the more the aging process speeds up.

Thus, getting older puts you in the inevitable position of having to mount ever stronger defenses against free radicals in futile attempts to beat the unbeatable. Eventually, of course, we all lose the battle to one thing or other. Which disease wounds you the deepest and finally mortally depends much on the shake of the genetic dice and your individual vulnerabilities.

As Dr. Harman puts it: "It is almost a matter of chance how life is terminated. If an organism does not die, for example, of cancer, it will soon die from some other rapidly developing disease, such as one of the cardiovascular system."

Aging is a disease. The human life span simply reflects the level of free radical oxidative damage that accumulates in cells. When enough damage accumulates, cells can't survive properly anymore and they just give up. —Earl R. Stadtman, researcher on aging, National Institutes of Health

Ultimately we are going to be able to get people to live a lot longer than anyone thinks. —Dr. Bruce N. Ames, University of California researcher and geneticist

HOW TO STOP THE DANCE OF DESTRUCTION

Now, obviously, since antioxidants can block, interrupt or repair the free radical rampages that promote aging, it makes sense to have a great deal of them around in your cells. The more that are present to protect cells' fragile membranes, proteins and genetic DNA, within toxic limits, the less able the free radicals are to strike and impose their damage. And the less damage, the less likely the telltale signs of aging and ultimate breakdown of the body. What's needed is a delicate balance—enough antioxidants to keep the free radicals under tight control so they cannot overrun the body, causing havoc. When you have far more free radicals than antioxidants in your system, you're in trouble, suffering what scientists call oxidant—another word for free radical—overload or stress. This imbalance nicks away at cells, setting the stage for accumulated damage that eventually becomes so severe we experience it as symptoms of one disease or other and overall aging.

Much aging, then, can be chalked up to a global

antioxidant deficiency—pitted against an environment, both internally and externally, rich in free radicals.

You get it. Run, don't walk, to find more antioxidants if you want to combat those rampaging free radicals that are stealing your youth.

Right off, there are three major ways to buck up your arsenal of antiaging antioxidants.

- ▲ The first obvious defense is to eat plenty of antioxidants, flooding your bloodstream and hence your cells with neutralizers of free radicals. This includes the powerful big three antioxidants—vitamin E, beta carotene and vitamin C—as well as more exotic antioxidants in supplements, herbs and foods such as garlic, broccoli, tea and tomatoes.
- ▲ Second, you can shun foods that are easily oxidized—chemically altered by ubiquitous oxygen so they generate free radicals inside your cells, wrecking them. Some prime examples are corn and safflower oil, margarine and dried eggs put in many processed foods.
- ▲ A third strategy is to ingest supplements, herbs, vitamins and other food constituents that indirectly stimulate enzymes to rev up the body's detoxification systems that zap free radicals. Notable is broccoli, which contains sulforaphane, a chemical that Johns Hopkins researchers recently found stimulates mechanisms that vaporize specific free radicals.

By feeding your cells antioxidants, you give them a powerful youth potion.

CHEMICAL DRAMA IN YOUR CELLS

What is a free radical? It is a molecule that has lost a vital piece of itself—one of its electrically charged electrons that orbit in pairs. To restore balance, the radical frantically steals an electron from nearby molecules or gives away the unpaired one. In so doing, it creates molecular mayhem, careening into the protein, fats and genetic DNA of cells, disfiguring and corroding them. If the target is fat, the radical can set off wildly destructive chain reactions that break down membranes, leaving cells to disintegrate. Upon meeting protein, the radical may shave off bits, destroying its ability to function. Hits on DNA, especially in the cells' tiny power factories called mitochondria, cause mutations that incite cells to aberrant behavior. Over time, the free radical damage takes its toll by leaving the body aged and diseased.

Enter the saviors—antioxidants. Simply, an antioxidant is a chemical that can donate a sought-after electron to a free radical without becoming dangerous itself. Thus an antioxidant, meeting a radical, puts an end to its rampage of cellular and bodily destruction—the slow degeneration known as aging.

THE FRISKY OLD FRUIT FLIES

How do scientists know that antioxidants can stop aging?

The proof is not total because the theory has not been, and probably never can be, tested on generations of humans. But many experiments with human cells and other species show the theory has biological validity. Consider, for example, a recent thrilling experiment on fruit flies that, some say, offers absolute proof of the free radical theory of aging.

If it can happen to fruit flies, it can happen to you.

Suppose you genetically altered a living creature so it produced more antioxidant enzymes to mop up free radicals. Now suppose such creatures lived longer and remained younger than identical creatures not treated to the antioxidant-bolstering gene. It would be pretty good proof that free radicals foster aging and that stronger antioxidant defenses slow down aging, says Earl Stadtman, chief of the laboratory of biochemistry at the National Heart, Lung and Blood Institute, and an authority on aging.

That's exactly what happened to fruit flies in groundbreaking experiments in 1994 by geneticists William Orr and Rajindar Sohal at Southern Methodist University in Dallas. Fruit flies genetically engineered to have souped-up antioxidant systems exceeded their normal life spans by one-third! Some even lived an unprecedented ninety-three days, setting a life span record for fruit flies.

More exciting, they carried their youthful vigor into old age. Scientists watching the tiny flies under magnifying glasses could instantly spot which had received the antioxidant-producing genes because they were "so much more vigorous." They walked 10 to 20 percent faster than normal flies their age. Halfway through life most could walk one centimeter per second—a brisk pace for a young fruit fly. "In other words, the quality of life of the flies was better. They were stronger physiologically," said Dr. Sohal.

This is not to suggest it's time to insert such genes in humans, but the experiment does dramatically prove the principle that an oversupply of antioxidant defenses in the body stretches life and vigor. For now, you must get antioxidants through your diet. But however they get into the cells of your body, they are apt to deter aging and prolong life. All life, after all, works on the same basic principles, says Dr. Harman. If antioxidants save fruit flies from earlier death and decrepitude, there's every reason to think they can do the same for you.

By the way, you can't actually consume the fruit flies' geriatric medicine. The experiment revved up superoxide dismutase (SOD) and catalase in the flies, major enzymes fueling the antioxidant machinery. Both SOD and catalase are sold in health food stores. But, unlike antioxidants in food, they do no good when eaten directly; they are simply destroyed in the gastric juices of the stomach and not absorbed.

New Memories for Geriatric Gerbils

Another landmark experiment by John Carney at the University of Kentucky and Robert Floyd at the Oklahoma Medical Research Foundation showed that antioxidants can reverse brain damage in aging gerbils, even restoring short-term memory, previously regarded as one of the few irretrievable losses of old age. At first, very old gerbils made more than twice as many mistakes negotiating a maze as young gerbils. The young animals averaged about four errors and the old ones around ten errors. But after injections of a chemical called phenylbutylnitrone, or PBN, that traps free radicals, the geriatric gerbils made a spectacular comeback, making only four errors, the same as the young ones. Moreover, examinations of the gerbils' brains revealed a biological reason for the memory rebirth: free radical damage to brain proteins had substantially diminished!

This indicates that free radical damage was responsible for memory loss and that free radical antagonists reversed it. It bodes well for humans, says Dr. Carney, because autopsies show that aged human brains, like those of gerbils, have much more oxidized damaged protein than the brains of young people.

NIH's Earl Stadtman was ecstatic: "The experiment marked the first time that a physiological function—the return of youthful brain chemistry and the restoration of short-term memory—has been clearly linked to the level of oxidized protein in the cell. The loss of memory with age can apparently be overcome."

Dr. Carney speculates that the PBN rejuvenates a system that is normally there when we are young but progressively declines as we get older. It suggests the thrilling possibility that the right antioxidants could not just prevent a failing memory, but bring it back. Further, Dr. Carney found, PBN animals were less likely to suffer brain damage after having a stroke.

Using the same PBN on mice, Dr. Richard Cutler, a research chemist with the National Institute on Aging's Gerontology Research Center in Baltimore, additionally prolonged the life span of older mice about 20 percent—comparable to giving fifteen more years to seventy-five-year-old humans. "It not only seems to slow down aging, but seems to reverse aging. This was unbelievable to me," said Cutler.

However, as Dr. Stadtman points out, the brain rejuvenation, sadly, was not permanent. When the injections of antioxidant PBN were discontinued, the gerbils' failing memory and poor maze performance returned. Thus, antioxidants for the elderly—and perhaps for everyone—may be somewhat like insulin for diabetics. There is no permanent antiaging fix. You must continuously feed your cells goodly amounts of antioxidants to try to keep the biological clock ticking as slowly as possible.

To be sure, you cannot outwit the aging process entirely to achieve immortality or even live past the built-in life span limits for our species, which many experts put at 120 years. Nor is there much wisdom in wanting to live longer than you are capable of enjoying it. The goal is not to simply stretch life span but to increase "functional" life span or "health span" in which your mind is alert and your body active. Science is bringing that promise closer than at any time in human history.

———

We could save billions of dollars if we could delay onset of chronic diseases by as little as ten years.
—Dr. Jeffrey Blumberg, Tufts, who advises adults to take antioxidant vitamin supplements

———

Strong Potions
from the
Fountain of Youth

Here's the equation that permits quantum leaps in your ability to combat aging:

▲ Free radicals damage cells, causing aging.
▲ Antioxidants block free radical damage.
▲ Thus, antioxidants help block aging.

Once you have an intellectual grip on that, the rest is clear:

▲ Find them.
▲ Use them.
▲ Stop aging.
▲ Stay young.
▲ Live longer.

There are more antiaging agents in the universe than you could ever dream of and probably more than science can discover in the next century. But many of these barriers to aging are here now, right in front of our faces in the form of vitamins, minerals, natural enzymes and amino acids, herbs, plants, foods and other natural substances.

Evidence is piling up, showing how they can fight aging. Prestigious medical journals are full of reports, unimagined ten years ago, documenting the awesome powers of such natural substances to prevent, halt and reverse the deterioration that comes with advancing years. The evidence comes from mainstream institutions such as Harvard, the University of California, Tufts, Johns Hopkins, Stanford, UCLA and Yale, among many.

The antiaging powers of some of the substances now being tested have been suspected for centuries, some for only a few years. Some of the names are familiar, such as vitamin E and C. Others are less so, such as ginkgo, coenzyme Q-10 and glutathione, just now emerging as superstars in the laboratories of scientists trying to slow down the aging process.

Consistently, research shows that the antiaging agents have antioxidant activity that helps delay onset of a diversity of aging diseases through a common pathway— warding off free radical damage to cells. Thus, many antioxidant substances such as vitamin E and vitamin C as well as coenzyme Q-10 may all work individually and together to prevent the same manifestations of aging, such as cancer, heart disease and brain degeneration.

As scientists understand more about the free radical theory of aging and how antioxidants can counteract it, it becomes ever more apparent that a unique and recently recognized deficiency of these natural substances generates our epidemic of premature and needless aging. Here, essentially, is what you need to know about the latest research on vitamins, minerals, herbs, foods and other natural substances in order to stay as young as possible as long as possible.

The Antiaging Vitamin Revolution

Why do you need vitamins and minerals, especially as you age? To save your arteries from destruction, your brain from vaporizing, your cells from cancer and your immune system from disappearing. Those are only a few of the reasons. The fact is, vitamins and minerals can help blunt some of the consequences of growing old. In fact, growing old itself—and the diseases that tag along—may be to a large extent an unrecognized vitamin deficiency disease of incredible magnitude! Thus, taking vitamins and minerals makes excellent sense. Indeed, in light of the mounting evidence, it seems reckless not to take them.

> **The argument can be made that we have set our standards of lifetime health and longevity far too low. When it comes to warding off chronic diseases and aging, everybody is in a sense deficient, or we would all live to our maximum potential.**

Welcome to the "vitamin revolution," or the "earthquakelike shift in the vitamin paradigm," as it's been variously described. No longer do scientists see vitamins and minerals as just the mundane stuff in food that builds strong bones and corrects deficiencies such as scurvy. "We are opening up a whole new frontier for vitamins," says vitamin investigator Dr. Ishwarlal Jialal, associate professor of internal medicine and clinical nutrition at the University of Texas Southwestern Medical Center at Dallas. In the new order of things, certain key vitamins in doses exceeding those in food promise protection against aging and disease far beyond all previous expectations. "Antioxidants such as vitamin C, vitamin E and beta carotene may prove as potent as antibiotics and vaccines in fighting disease," declares vitamin C investigator Dr. Matthias Rath, a colleague of the late Linus Pauling. "The evidence that these pills can be beneficial is overwhelming," says Earl Stadtman, biochemist and aging expert at the National Heart, Lung and Blood Institute.

Indeed, the accumulating evidence is staggering.

The case for taking vitamins and minerals grows so persuasive that not taking them is an invitation to reckless aging and premature death. Numerous studies show that people who take vitamins delay the onset and severity of aging diseases.

▲ People who take vitamins, especially vitamin C and vitamin E, live several years longer than people who don't.

▲ Faltering immune systems as you age can be rejuvenated by taking vitamins, sometimes a simple multiple-vitamin pill.

▲ Heart disease victims have comparatively low blood and tissue levels of dietary antioxidants, including vitamin E, vitamin C, beta carotene and selenium.

▲ Those most susceptible to cancer also have comparatively low blood and tissue levels of dietary antioxidants, including vitamin E, vitamin C, beta carotene and selenium.

▲ A deficiency in B vitamins can trigger senility, artery damage, heart attack and some cancers; replenishing the vitamins often prevents or remedies these problems.

▲ A marginal chromium deficiency can precipitate a midlife slide into diabetes and cardiovascular disease.

▲ Calcium and vitamin D supplements after a year

can dramatically prevent broken bones even in eighty-year-olds.

▲ Regularly taking any type of vitamin slashes the odds of common skin cancer 70 percent, Johns Hopkins investigators report.

▲ Regular vitamin takers have a 27 percent lower risk of developing cataracts, say Harvard researchers.

THE FRONTIER BEYOND FOOD

Bothersome philosophical question: If we need heavy doses of vitamins and minerals, why didn't nature put them in food in the first place? Isn't it unnatural to take supra-natural doses in pills? No.

Fast disappearing is the dogma that food can give you everything you need to get through the tough years of old age. This is not to fault nature for deliberately short-changing us. Maybe she didn't foresee the hazards modern civilization would bring. Some scientists think we simply need more antioxidant vitamins and minerals to stay even with the aging process because we are exposed to increased barrages from our polluted environment, including pesticides, radiation from nuclear energy, auto exhaust, smog, fat and chemical-loaded processed foods— all of which step up the free radical attacks on our bodies and thus cause us to age prematurely. In this new self-created hazardous landscape or "unnatural environment," we require "heroic countermeasures" in the form of antioxidant vitamins and minerals to boost our biological defenses and survival odds, says vitamin C champion Emanuel Cheraskin, M.D., emeritus professor of medicine at the University of Alabama.

ANTIAGING SECRETS OF THE EXPERTS

Earl Stadtman, Ph.D., age seventy-five:
Pioneering Biochemist
Chief of the Laboratory of Biochemistry,
National Heart, Lung and Blood Institute

Dr. Stadtman is a well-known authority on free radicals and has done much research demonstrating that aging is characterized by an accumulation of cell damage from free radical attacks.

"I think of aging as a disease—a process of progressive physical or mental debilitation, and one of the important elements responsible is the generation of free radicals. Anything that increases the rate of free radical damage contributes to the aging process."

Here's what he takes daily to delay aging:

▲ Vitamin E—400 IU.
▲ Vitamin C—500 milligrams.
▲ Beta carotene—25,000 IU.

Another view is that we need the extra vitamins and minerals in a sense to outwit nature and stay around much longer than intended. We were never meant to so effectively defeat infections early in life as we now do with antibiotics and hang around so long, racking up the accumulated damage to cells and propelling so many of us into old age, believes aging expert Dr. Denham Harman. He thinks nature's intent is to dump us after middle age when we have completed our procreation duties. To survive longer in good health, he says, we need the extra boost from antioxidants, including megadoses of vitamins and minerals. After all, "from an evolutionary point of view, passing on genes to the next generation is what matters, not a long and biologically useless old age," as *New Scientist* magazine aptly put it.

"Nature originally designed humans to live about thirty years—the time needed to reach sexual maturation and raise children to independence," says Leonard Hayflick, professor of anatomy at the University of California San Francisco School of Medicine and author of *How and Why We Age.*

Wearing a seat belt doesn't give you a license to drive recklessly, it just protects you in case of an accident. Vitamin supplements work the same way: they don't give you a license to eat poorly and otherwise abuse your health, but provide an added cushion of protection. —Dr. Jeffrey Blumberg, Tufts University

---

THE RDAS ARE POOR PROTECTION

If you strive for ordinary poor health, some experts joke, follow the RDAs—or recommended dietary allowances— figures touted by government officials as the amount of vitamins and minerals necessary to prevent common deficiency diseases such as scurvy and rickets. But if you want optimum health, aim higher—ten to two hundred times higher than the RDAs. That's what many experts now urge. Tufts professor Jeffrey Blumberg considers the RDAs "increasingly irrelevant to today's public health concerns of aging and chronic disease." The RDAs do not pretend to address prevention of heart disease, cancer, cataracts, arthritis and other age-related diseases, he points out.

Dr. Linus Pauling once called vitamin supplements a technological advance that can usher in a new era of optimal health, not merely survival. Vitamin megadoses can prime the body's cells to perform at their genetic peak of efficiency, he argued, slowing the aging process and minimizing degenerative diseases.

But most Americans do not even meet the standards of vitamin intake for basic survival, let alone optimum health. Deficiencies in the bare minimum set by the RDAs are widespread in older Americans, underscoring how dismal the situation is as we approach the prime time for the appearance of chronic diseases. Tufts researcher on aging Dr. Robert Russell notes that "almost no one" ages sixty-five to seventy-five meets the RDA requirements, poor as they are. Most older Americans do not even get two-thirds of the RDAs for many of the critical B vitamins and vitamin C.

Further, standards of measuring deficiencies are old-fashioned and irrelevant. Ordinary blood tests are not an adequate measure of vitamin status. You can have "normal" blood levels of vitamins and still be metabolically deficient, meaning you lack the amount needed for normal biological activity. According to a new concept, you can also have a "localized" vitamin deficiency, in which your blood tests normal, but cells in specific tissues, for example, in the lung or cervix, are deficient, exposing you to a greater risk of cancer and possibly other chronic maladies.

THE ALARMING FACTS

▲ Half of all Americans past sixty are deficient even by minimum standards in vitamin E, vitamin C and vitamin A or beta carotene, according to Tufts researchers.

▲ As you age, your vitamins run out of steam. You need more just to stay even. Many physiological changes and chronic disease risks attributed to age are actually caused by higher demands for vitamins.

▲ Heart disease, cancer, arthritis, diabetes and cataracts are really "accelerated aging," tied to widespread vitamin-mineral deficiencies or "insufficiencies," as some scientists now term it.

Vitamins and minerals are here to help save you from the diseases of growing old. In fact, growing old itself—and the diseases that tag along—are to a large extent a vitamin deficiency disease of incredible magnitude.

WHAT YOU NEED TO KNOW ABOUT VITAMINS TO FEND OFF AGING

▲ Think of aging and its consequences as partly a vitamin-mineral "deficiency disease" of global proportions.

▲ To best stave off aging, it's necessary to take megadoses of antioxidant vitamins and minerals, notably vitamin E, vitamin C and beta carotene.

▲ It's no longer smart to think food can give you all the vitamins and minerals you need to interfere with aging.

▲ The role of vitamins and minerals is not just to stave off obvious deficiency diseases such as scurvy and rickets. They are also warriors against our chronic age-driven epidemic of heart disease and cancer.

▲ You can't rely on the government-sanctioned recommended modest doses of vitamins and minerals (RDAs) to combat the ravages of aging to the maximum, although sometimes even small amounts can reverse age-related deterioration.

▲ Know you are probably deficient even in the minimal RDA requirements for vitamins and minerals. Nearly all Americans are. Thus, you are flirting dangerously with premature aging.

▲ The main way vitamins and minerals combat aging is by boosting antioxidant activity, helping crush the free radicals that are a prime cause of aging.

▲ Many vitamins and minerals also help keep the lid on other physiological processes that promote aging, hence disease, disability and death.

▲ Contrary to what you sometimes hear, vitamins and minerals in antiaging doses are remarkably safe and free of side effects.

▲ Vitamins and minerals are cheap, especially compared with the enormity of good they do and the money they save in drugs, high-tech procedures, doctor's bills and hospitalization.

▲ Numerous vitamins and minerals work together to protect against aging. There is no one antiaging miracle vitamin or mineral. "A number of studies show that antioxidants work better in combination than individually," says Dr. Carl Cotman, director of the Irvine Brain Aging Unit of the University of California.

LOOK WHAT HAPPENS TO PEOPLE
WHO TAKE ANTIOXIDANTS

Death Rates: Down 50 Percent: National Institute on Aging researchers recently found that taking both vitamin C and vitamin E pills chopped death risk from any cause in half among ten thousand elderly persons, ages 67 to 105. Further, the elderly vitamin takers had only one-third as many heart disease deaths as non–vitamin takers.

Cancer Deaths: Down 13 Percent: The most dramatic proof that taking antioxidant vitamins can cut cancer and cancer deaths comes from a 1993 National Cancer Institute study in Linxian County, China. In the study of nearly thirty thousand people over age forty, vitamins slashed deaths in those who took daily doses of 15 milligrams of beta carotene, 30 milligrams of vitamin E and 50 micrograms of selenium. In only five years, deaths from all causes dropped 9 percent. Most significant was an overall fall in cancer deaths of 13 percent. Specifically, esophageal cancer deaths fell 4 percent, stomach cancer deaths 21 percent and lung cancer deaths 45 percent. Rates of all other cancers decreased 20 percent. Deaths from strokes also fell 10 percent. Of high interest, investigators noticed a drop in cancer deaths incredibly quickly—within one to two years after subjects started taking antioxidants. Presumably the antioxidants worked by guarding cells from free radical damage.

Cancer Survival: Up 50 Percent: Equally impressive, vitamin megadoses can help fight existing cancer. In a recent study by Dr. Donald Lamm, head of urology at West Virginia University in Morgantown, vitamin supplements "dramatically" cut the recurrence of bladder cancer in half and nearly doubled the survival time of patients. In the study, sixty-five patients all took a standard immunotherapy drug called BCG. About half also got high daily doses of antioxidant vitamins (40,000 IU of vitamin A, 100 milligrams of B6, 2,000 milligrams of vitamin C, 400 IU of vitamin E and 90 milligrams of zinc). After nearly two years, 40 percent who took the vitamins plus the drug developed new tumors compared with 80 percent taking only the drug. Most probably, says Dr. Lamm, the supplements worked by boosting immune defenses. Such anticancer therapy should be monitored by a physician.

Heart Attacks, Strokes: Down 50 Percent: About twenty-two thousand male physicians are taking 50 milligrams of beta carotene every other day as part of a long-term double-blind Harvard study. Recently, investigators analyzed data from a subgroup of 333 physicians who had signs of heart disease, such as angina (chest pain). The surprising finding: Those on beta carotene for six years suffered only half as many heart attacks, strokes, bypass surgeries and cardiac deaths as doctors taking a dummy pill. Note: The protection kicked in after only two years.

More evidence: Men who said they took vitamins, mainly vitamin E, over a ten-year period, had 78 percent fewer heart disease deaths, 58 percent fewer heart attacks, 15 percent less angina and 40 percent fewer first-time cardiac "events" than non–vitamin takers. The study of 2,226 men was done at Laval University in Quebec. The U.S. government's First National Health and Nutrition Examination Survey found that Americans who regularly took vitamin C supplements had 37 percent fewer fatal heart attacks.

Skin Cancer: Down 70 Percent: Just regularly taking vitamin supplements in general, but particularly vitamins A, C and E, slashed the risk of our most common cancer—basal cell carcinoma, a skin cancer—by an astonishing 70 percent, according to a 1994 study at Johns Hopkins University. If applied to the entire aging population, vitamins thus might prevent 350,000 new cases of basal cell carcinoma a year, researchers said.

Immunity Up, Infections Down: 50 Percent: A simple one-a-day multiple-vitamin pill, Theragran-M, boosted immune functions significantly in older healthy people with good diets who had no signs of deficiencies, according to a study at the New Jersey Medical School. In another groundbreaking study by Ranjit K. Chandra at Memorial University in Newfoundland, a combination of eighteen vitamins and minerals in mostly modest doses slashed infectious illnesses in older people nearly in half within a year's time.

Cataracts: Down 27 to 36 Percent: Men taking a multivitamin pill were only 73 percent as likely to develop cataracts as non–vitamin takers, according to a Harvard Medical School study of seventeen thousand male physicians past age forty-five. Also, in the National Cancer Institute's Linxian, China, study, some subjects took a combination of twenty-six vitamins and minerals in moderate doses, about one and a half to three times higher than the RDA. The rate of nuclear cataracts in those vitamin takers over age sixty-five dropped 36 percent.

NATURAL REJUVENATORS AND LONGEVITY TONICS

Familiar vitamins and minerals are by no means the only natural substances with antioxidant, antiaging, disease-preventing and disease-alleviating powers. Numerous plants and natural extracts are full of antioxidants and other biologically active chemicals. Antiaging substances abound in the leaves, stems and roots of countless edible and inedible plants. Many have been used as medicinal herbs for thousands of years. Indeed, at least one-fourth of our prescription drugs are derived from plants.

Also, there's an amazing new scientific realization that as the body's internally produced supplies of antiaging enzymes, hormones, amino acids and other natural protections run down as we grow older, we can synthesize identical biological clones and use them to replenish the shortages, thus rejuvenating tissues and restoring youthful vigor—sometimes to an astonishing degree. Just because time depletes our internally generated defenses does not mean we must abandon all hope of building them back up again. We do not need to go quietly and unprotesting into aging.

Undeniably, you can use many of nature's substances in addition to vitamins and minerals to help stave off the ravages of aging. Physicians in Europe and Japan often prescribe such substances—for example, the herb ginkgo can help reverse declining mental abilities and energy *before the more dramatic consequences of aging set in*. Another widely used natural substance in many other European countries, as well as Japan, is coenzyme Q-10, a vitaminlike chemical produced by the body in smaller quantities as you age. An antioxidant, it helps heart cells, in particular, function more efficiently as you age, perhaps postponing the day your heart goes into failure.

THE GARDEN OF ETERNITY

Nothing keeps your cells young, vibrant and disease-resistant like eating lots of fruits and vegetables. They are powerful antidotes to growing old, infirm and disease-burdened. Antioxidant authority Dr. Bruce Ames bluntly says, "If you don't eat your veggies, you're really irradiating yourself," exposing yourself to needless cell destruction and cancer. University of Minnesota's Dr. John Potter ties our cancer epidemic to a widespread "vegetable deficiency." Studies consistently show that eating five or more servings of fruits and vegetables daily can cut your cancer risk in half and save your life in other ways.

Death rates dropped 28 percent in men who ate a carrot's worth of beta carotene and two and a half oranges worth of vitamin C every day. Cancer deaths also fell 50 percent and heart disease deaths 18 percent over a twenty-four-year period, investigators at the University of Texas School of Public Health in Houston documented. A recent study in Finland found that cardiovascular deaths sank as people took in more antioxidants E, C and carotenoids from fruits and vegetables. All fruits and vegetables are carriers of vast quantities of known and unknown antioxidants.

Indeed, in Germany and Japan, the government has designed regulatory mechanisms for approving the use of such natural inedible and edible substances to prevent and alleviate diseases. Not surprisingly, much of the scientific research on natural agents to retard aging and prolong life has been done in Germany and Japan. However, many researchers at prominent scientific institutions in the United States now have also joined in, confirming the validity of such research. Some elite academicians, such as Bruce Ames, Lester Packer and others at the University of California in Berkeley, are directing their investigations toward antioxidants produced internally by the body, such as ubiquinol (coenzyme Q-10,) and antioxidant herbs, such as ginkgo. Nevertheless, all may help save your cells from free radical damage and aging and, like vitamins, are available at health food stores and are increasingly being prescribed by doctors.

ANTIAGING, LIFE-STRETCHING SUPERFOODS

What you eat every day, starting when you are young and extending over a lifetime, has a profound and everlasting impact on your survival, health, aging and longevity. Foods are chemical concoctions of awesome complexity that enter your cells, altering their composition and dictating their activity. Although you may not think of them as such, foods are potent packages of pharmacological agents that control the behavior of your cells. What you give your cells can make them fortresses filled with armies of antioxidants to resist the ravages of time and free radical attacks that are the primary cause of aging and age-related diseases. Or you can provide foods devoid of antioxidants, allowing wholesale massacres and mutilation of your cells—diminishing your prospects for delayed aging and longevity.

As your cells age, so does your body. And how fast your cells age depends greatly on whether you give them antioxidant-rich foods or antioxidant-poor and free radical–rich foods.

Some foods are undoubtedly endowed with thousands of antioxidants and other agents that bolster antioxidant activity. Nobody knows the exact antioxidant composition of such foods because they have not been completely chemically dissected and may never be. So far, however, scientists have discovered amazing antioxidant activity in many fruits, vegetables, legumes, grains and oils. Further, hundreds of studies linking diet and disease identify strong antiaging, antidisease foods.

The Vitamin You *Must* Take to Delay Aging

▲ ▲ ▲

(Why You Need Vitamin E to Stop Aging)

If you take no other vitamins, take vitamin E. It's virtually impossible to get heart disease–fighting, cancer-fighting, immune-boosting doses of vitamin E from food—unless you eat more than 5,000 calories a day, most of them in fat.

Vitamin E is the Michael Jordan–super defense against aging—the radical-fighting antioxidant you want on your side above all others. When you ask top-gun researchers around the world which vitamin supplement is most crucial to scare off the diseases of aging, the choice is almost universally vitamin E, also called alpha tocopherol. And with good reason. The age-fighting effects of vitamin E in supra-food doses are becoming legendary. Indeed, the startling new evidence about vitamin E has done more than anything else to shake doctors' faith in the old dictum that you can get all the life-preserving help you need from food. Vitamin E supplements seem necessary to combat the aging problems of modern civilization.

HOW VITAMIN E CAN FIGHT AGING

Blocks Artery Clogging: Vitamin E fights our greatest aging fear, atherosclerosis, the gradual clogging and hardening of arteries that begins in youth, worsens in middle age and kills about half a million Americans a year, primarily in old age. New thinking: Atherosclerosis occurs in large part because bad-type LDL blood cholesterol is chemically altered—oxidized or turned rancid and toxic—by free radical attacks. If such LDL oxidation does not occur, bad LDL cholesterol is not able to infiltrate artery walls, the first step to plaque buildup and artery clogging. Thus, blocking such oxidation or "rancidity" of LDL cholesterol nips the clogging, narrowing and disintegration of arteries in the bud. That's what antioxidant vitamin E supplements do expertly—far better than any other antioxidant vitamin. Vitamin E enters the LDL cholesterol molecule and inhibits hazardous oxidation, thus switching off the very genesis of coronary heart disease.

A study by Ishwarlal Jialal of the University of Texas Southwestern Medical Center in Dallas found that taking 800 IU of vitamin E a day for three months slashed LDL cholesterol oxidation—and thus its ability to foster artery damage and heart disease—a dramatic 40 percent! "It's very clear that vitamin E is the most potent antioxidant against LDL oxidation," he says. He found it takes at least 400 IU of vitamin E per day to significantly prevent LDL cholesterol from being oxidized.

Zaps Heart Attacks: The scientific community was wowed by two recent large-scale Harvard studies, both showing that taking vitamin E supplements seems to dramatically reduce the appearance of heart disease. First in women: Among eighty-seven thousand nurses, incidents of major heart disease was 41 percent lower in those who reported taking from 100 to 250 IU daily of vitamin E pills for more than two years compared with those who did not take vitamin E supplements. Such vitamin-takers also had a 29

VITAMIN E REJUVENATES OLD ARTERIES

In monkeys, 108 IU of vitamin E daily for three years slowed down and reversed artery blockage due to a high-fat diet, according to research at the University of Mississippi's Atherosclerosis Research Laboratory. Animals were fed a high-fat diet; those that also got vitamin E had only one-fifth as much artery blockage as monkeys denied vitamin E. More amazing, in monkeys with established artery disease, vitamin E actually cleared arteries of plaque by about 60 percent. The blockages shrank from an average 35 percent artery closure to a 15 percent closure in two years!

Vitamin E seems to have the same potential in humans, according to research by Howard N. Hodis at the University of Southern California School of Medicine, who found that vitamin E appeared to retard and slightly reverse arterial plaque formation in middle-aged men undergoing coronary bypass surgery. Men who reported taking at least 100 IU of vitamin E daily (along with other medication) had less narrowed arteries after two years than those taking less vitamin E. More spectacular, angiograms (X rays) revealed that the plaque in the arteries of some vitamin E takers had shrunk, signifying an actual regression in atherosclerosis!

percent lower stroke risk and a decrease in overall mortality rates of 13 percent.

Men were saved, too. Among forty thousand middle-aged men, those taking more than 100 IU of vitamin E a day for more than two years showed a 37 percent lower risk of major cardiovascular mishaps, including heart attacks. Vitamin E does not work overnight. The Harvard research suggests you must take vitamin E for at least two years before heart attack protection kicks in.

Important fact: Harvard authors Meir J. Stampfer, M.D., and Eric B. Rimm, Sc.D., stressed that you can't get enough vitamin E in food to suppress heart attacks. That requires vitamin E supplements, which both authors take. However, more than 250 IU a day did not additionally cut heart disease in their study.

Question: Can you afford *not* to take vitamin E?

Answer: The penalty may be harsh, if the Harvard study is accurate. "The risk for not taking vitamin E was equivalent to the risk of smoking," marveled Dr. Rimm.

In fact, the study indicated that the benefits of taking vitamin E far exceeded the benefits seen from reducing high blood pressure and high cholesterol! A large World Health Organization study of men in sixteen European cities agreed that high blood levels of vitamin E are more apt to prevent fatal heart attacks than lowering blood cholesterol is.

Rejuvenates Immunity: Dr. Simin Meydani, a nutritional immunologist at Tufts University, tested vitamin E supplements (doses of either 400 or 800 IU a day) on people over age sixty. Their immune responses had been declining with age, but shot back up, "almost to the level of young people," she said. Although the vitamin did not work in every person, in most, the recharge of immunity was phenomenal. Immune functions, such as proliferation of white blood cells that fight infections, jumped by 10 to 50 percent within thirty days! Some functions improved as much as 80 to 90 percent.

Rationale: Dr. Meydani believes vitamin E helps guard the fat in membranes of immune cells from being oxidized by free radical attacks. Such cells are particularly vulnerable to free radical damage. Note: These subjects were not deficient in vitamin E by current standards. To rejuvenate immune functions, older people need supplement boosts of vitamin E far beyond "normal" requirements. Vitamin E megadoses boosted immune functioning in young people too, but not as much as in older people.

Thwarts Cancer: A recent study of thirty-five thousand Iowa women found that those under age sixty-five who got the most vitamin E—largely from supplements—had a 68 percent lower chance of colon cancer. Low blood levels of vitamin E make you 50 percent more susceptible to all kinds of cancers, a large Finnish study concluded. Taking vitamin E for six months cut the risk of cancers of the mouth and throat in half, according to National Cancer Institute researchers. In another study, taking vitamin E supplements cut lung cancer risk in half among nonsmokers, according to Yale University researchers. The anticancer effect is attributed mostly to vitamin E's immune-boosting feats. However, there is new evidence that vitamin E directly inhibits growth of cancer cells.

Relieves Arthritis: In a few studies, doses up to 1,200 milligrams of vitamin E was as effective as a common anti-inflammatory drug at relieving pain, swelling and morning stiffness caused by rheumatoid arthritis. Speculation: Arthritics often have low blood levels of vitamin E—and may need extra amounts, because it is rapidly consumed trying to fight off free radical inflammatory attacks on joints.

We have hundreds of thousands of people dying in this country from heart disease and cancer. I think

*the evidence suggesting vitamin E can reduce the suf-
fering and costs of these diseases is very strong and
there appears to be no downside. Vitamin E doesn't
even cost much.* —Dr. Jeffrey Blumberg, chief of the
Antioxidant Research Laboratory at Tufts University

Postpones Cataracts: Vitamin E can arrest and reverse
development of cataracts in laboratory animals. In
humans, one study found that taking vitamin E supplements pushed the risk down by 56 percent, although vitamin C was more powerful.

Retards Overall Brain and Blood Aging: Over time free
radical damage leaves footprints in cells—a buildup of a
substance called lipofuscin, also called the aging pigment.
Levels of this aging pigment fell significantly in certain
cells of older patients who took vitamin E. Blood circulation in their brains also improved. Some scientists believe
vitamin E may help delay age-related loss of mental faculties, including that from Alzheimer's disease.

*Adults should take 100 to 400 IU (international
units) of vitamin E a day!* —The Alliance for Aging
Research, a Washington-based nonprofit organization
on aging research

How Does It Work? Vitamin E is a very powerful fat-
soluble antioxidant, hence able to do its best work in the
fattiest parts of the anatomy. Vitamin E appears especially
critical in preventing brain, artery and immune system
deterioration because the brain and immune cell mem-

THE ANTIAGING PROMISE OF VITAMIN E

- ▲ Stops free radical chain reactions that destroy cells.
- ▲ Blocks oxidation of detrimental LDL cholesterol and other cell-damaging fats.
- ▲ Prevents heart attacks and strokes.
- ▲ Keeps arteries from clogging.
- ▲ Rejuvenates immunity.
- ▲ Prevents cancer and blocks growth of cancer cells.
- ▲ Protects the brain from degenerative diseases.
- ▲ Relieves arthritis symptoms.
- ▲ Fights cataracts and macular degeneration.
- ▲ Relieves intermittent claudication, decreased blood flow to leg arteries.

branes are very fatty and arteries are extremely susceptible to damage from fat. Specifically, vitamin E acts like a little fire extinguisher to snuff out chains of ferocious free radical attacks that turn fat in your brain and blood rancid, disturbing normal functioning and making your tissues age faster.

What About Food? Because vitamin E is fat-soluble, it's concentrated in fatty foods, such as vegetable oils (primarily soybean, sunflower and corn oils), nuts and seeds, whole grains and wheat germs. It's also in some vegetables. But it's virtually impossible to get age-retarding doses of vitamin E in food. To get 400 IU—a typical capsule dose—Dr. Alan Chait, heart disease researcher at the University of Washington, points out you would have to drink two quarts of corn oil or eat more than five pounds of wheat germ, eight cups of almonds or twenty-eight cups of peanuts. The peanuts contain 22,520 calories and 1,912 grams of fat. The most you can expect from food alone is about 25 IU daily. Dr. Chait takes no chances. He takes a vitamin E supplement.

Do You Need a Supplement? Absolutely yes if you want extra protection against aging, since you can't get antiaging doses from food. And you need a separate supplement because you cannot get enough in a typical multivitamin-mineral pill, which contains about 30 IU of vitamin E.

How Much? You need at least 100 IU of vitamin E daily to get any measurable protection against heart attacks, studies show. However, a preferred dose is 400 IU of vitamin E because that much is needed to block dangerous LDL cholesterol oxidation, a prerequisite for artery clogging. That dose also boosts immunity. Take vitamin E with meals. If possible, take a couple of doses during the day rather than a single large dose to keep blood levels consistently high.

What Type? Natural vitamin E or synthetic? In dry form or in oil-based capsules? It makes little difference, say many experts. The most biologically active form of vitamin E is known as alpha tocopherol. A *d* before alpha tocopherol means it's from natural sources—a *dl* means it's synthetic. New research finds that the cheaper synthetic type (dl-alpha tocopherol) blocks dangerous oxidation of LDL cholesterol just as well as natural vitamin E or d-alpha tocopherol does. However, some researchers still regard natural vitamin E as superior.

How Much Is Too Much? Most experts consider daily doses of 400 to 800 IU very safe, with no known toxic effects. Indeed, a one-year study of eight hundred patients found no adverse effects from a daily dose of 2,000 IU of vitamin E. However, in doses exceeding 400 IU, vitamin E, like aspirin, does have mild anticlotting activity, "thinning the blood," and is not recommended in people taking anticoagulant drugs or facing surgery. Toxicity can occur at over 3,200 IU daily; signs include headaches, diarrhea and elevated blood pressure. "Don't take more than 1,000 IU daily," advises vitamin E expert Dr. Ishwarlal Jialal.

Caution: If you are taking anticoagulants, or suspect any type of bleeding problem, check with your doctor before taking vitamin E. It can have an anticoagulant effect.

In a recent Finnish study, vitamin E may have contributed to hemorrhagic or "bleeding stroke" in smokers, although most experts believe that the 50-IU dose used was too low to alter blood coagulation or to have other beneficial or detrimental effects.

Your Best Vitamin for Longevity

▲   ▲   ▲

(Why You Need Vitamin C to Stop Aging)

If you want to live longer, eat lots of fruits and vegetables and take vitamin C pills, starting now! "A thirty-five-year-old man who eats vitamin C–rich foods and takes vitamin C supplements will slash his chances of heart disease death by two-thirds and live 6.3 years longer," predicts Dr. James Enstrom, UCLA researcher. "We could add an extra twelve to eighteen years to our lives by taking from 3,200 to 12,000 milligrams of vitamin C a day," claimed the late Dr. Linus Pauling.

Two-time Nobel Prize–winning scientist Dr. Linus Pauling died of cancer in 1994 at age ninety-three. But he fervently believed he had delayed his departure by at least twenty years by taking vitamins for half a century, notably extravagant megadoses of vitamin C, which he passionately insisted could help overcome disease and prolong life. Mounting evidence suggests he was right. New studies from the nation's bastions of mainstream medicine now indicate that even low doses of vitamin C can give your life expectancy a quantum boost.

"We've now got the first solid proof that vitamin C can add years to your life," says Morton A. Klein, who with UCLA's James E. Enstrom, Ph.D., analyzed government data on the dietary intakes of eleven thousand Americans. Indeed, they found that getting about 300 milligrams of vitamin C daily (roughly half in supplements) added six years to a man's life and two years to a woman's life. "Deaths from cardiovascular disease alone dropped by over 40 percent in the male vitamin C takers," declares Klein. The remarkable life-prolonging benefits from vitamin C far outstrip what you can expect from lowering your cholesterol and cutting down on fat, argues Dr. Enstrom. Further, vitamin C takers lived longer despite smoking, overweight, lack of exercise and even poor diets.

Like the vast majority of Americans, you may have an unsuspected, invisible vitamin C deficiency that is needlessly robbing you of youth, optimum health and longevity. Emanuel Cheraskin, M.D., emeritus professor of medicine at the University of Alabama and vitamin C researcher, says: "Virtually nobody gets enough vitamin C."

THE ALARMING FACTS

▲ One-fourth of Americans do not get even the minimal rock-bottom amount of 60 milligrams of vitamin C that cells need to perform basic biological functions.

▲ Only 9 percent of Americans eat five daily fruits and vegetables (200 to 300 milligrams of vitamin C), urged by the National Cancer Institute.

▲ About 20 percent of healthy older people and 68 percent of elderly nonhospitalized patients had white blood cells deficient in vitamin C, according to one study.

HOW VITAMIN C CAN FIGHT AGING

Immunizes Against Cancer: Overwhelmingly, some 120 studies identify vitamin C as a form of vaccination against cancer. Consistently, people who take in the most vitamin C are only half as likely as the skimpiest vitamin C eaters to develop cancer, in particular cancers of the stomach, esophagus, pancreas and oral cavity, and possibly cervix, rectum and breast, according to analyses by Gladys Block, Ph.D., cancer epidemiologist at the University of California, Berkeley. Five daily servings of fruits and vegetables contain 200 to 300 milligrams of vitamin C—enough to help retard cancer. But for extra cancer insurance, you need a supplement. Dr. Block takes 2,000 to 3,000 milligrams of vitamin C a day.

Saves Arteries: Vitamin C offers wholesale protection of arteries. Surprisingly, modest amounts of vitamin C can drive up good-type HDL cholesterol that discourages artery clogging, reduce bad-type LDL cholesterol that destroys arteries, lower high blood pressure, strengthen blood vessel walls, make blood less sticky and thwart cholesterol-inspired changes leading to clogged arteries. People who get less vitamin C than in a daily orange averaged 11 mm/Hg higher systolic (upper number) and 6 mm/Hg higher diastolic pressure in studies by Paul Jacques at Tufts. Good HDLs were also the highest in women getting three oranges' worth of vitamin C daily and in men getting the C in five oranges, USDA tests showed. Most apt to respond were older people and men. Taking 600 milligrams of vitamin C or more a day also has made blood less sticky, thus less apt to form clots.

Most remarkably, vitamin C, like vitamin E, helps keep arteries young, clear and flexible by blocking the conversion of LDL cholesterol in your blood to a toxic type that clings to artery walls. In monkeys, moderate doses of vitamin C as well as E actually slowed down artery clogging and helped clear arteries damaged by high-fat diets.

ANTIAGING SECRETS OF THE EXPERTS

Linus Pauling, Ph.D.:
Nobel Laureate and Vitamin C Crusader

Just before he died at age ninety-three, Dr. Pauling said: "I have to attribute my health at this point largely to my intake of vitamins and minerals." Although he died of cancer, he believed vitamins had delayed the onset of the cancer by about twenty years. He claimed to have had no colds since he began taking high doses of vitamin C in 1965. He started taking a single vitamin pill in 1941. Later, he took 18,000 milligrams of vitamin C daily.

Dr. Pauling believed we could live an extra twelve to eighteen years if we took from 3,200 to 12,000 milligrams of vitamin C a day—the amount in 45 to 170 oranges.

Raises Immunity: A prime way your body revs up to fight foreign invaders, such as infectious bacteria and viruses, is to rally armies of white blood cells called lymphocytes. Taking 5,000 milligrams of vitamin C daily increased production of lymphocytes, and 10,000 milligrams increased production even more, according to National Cancer Institute researchers. Vitamin C has great influence on the cellular soldiers of the immune system. Dr. Cheraskin says the vitamin works like an antibiotic against bacteria.

Moreover, vitamin C dramatically boosts immune functioning by hiking the body's levels of the antioxidant glutathione, essential for proper immune functioning. When men in a U.S. Department of Agriculture study ate less than one-third the RDA for vitamin C for nine weeks, their glutathione blood levels plunged 50 percent. Even a slight deficiency in vitamin C could cause the body's immune defenses to plummet, researchers concluded. Five hundred milligrams of vitamin C a day boosted glutathione in red blood cells by 50 percent.

Reverses Biological Clock: British researchers have shown that vitamin C can actually reverse aging—by biochemically rejuvenating white blood cells in the elderly. In one study of older people, average age seventy-six, only 120 milligrams of vitamin C a day jacked up their white blood cell levels to equal those in the young, average age thirty-five, in just two weeks. In another remarkable double-blind study, only 30 to 50 milligrams a day of vitamin C did the same thing in elderly hospitalized patients. But this time their leukocytes became biochemically younger than those of the young subjects!.

Improves Sperm and Restores Male Fertility: Men with low levels of vitamin C are more likely to have defective sperm that could cause birth defects in offspring. In a landmark test at the University of California at Berkeley, free radical damage to the genetic material DNA doubled in the sperm cells of men restricted to 5 milligrams of vitamin C daily (the amount in a teaspoon of lemon juice). When the men returned to a daily diet with either 60 milligrams or 250 milligrams of vitamin C, the DNA damage to sperm declined within a month. That means eating a single orange a day could heal sperm and prevent male-induced birth defects in nonsmoking men. In other tests at the University of Texas, infertility was reversed in men who took at least 200 milligrams of vitamin C daily.

Prevents Lung Disease: Your lungs function better when you get lots of vitamin C. People who ate foods with 300 milligrams of vitamin C a day were only 70 percent as likely to have chronic bronchitis or asthma as those eating about 100 milligrams, according to a study of nine thousand adults by Dr. Joel Schwartz of the U.S. Environmental Protection Agency. Further, vitamin C helps stop leukocytes, white blood cells, from clumping and sticking to the walls of blood vessels—a characteristic of emphysema as well as atherosclerosis.

Combats Gum Disease: Lots of evidence suggests vitamin C fends off destructive free radical attacks on gum tissue. A recent study in Finland found periodontal disease— bleeding gums, deep pockets and receding gums—three and a half times more common in people with low blood levels of vitamin C.

Prevents Cataracts: Cataract victims are only 30 percent as likely to have taken vitamin C supplements as those who remain cataract-free, Canadian tests show.

Our Stone Age forefathers ate about 400 milligrams a day of vitamin C by foraging for wild greens and fruit. That means normal, healthy people should get at least that much. —Dr. Emanuel Cheraskin, University of Alabama

Adults should take 250 to 1,000 milligrams of vitamin C supplements a day. —The Alliance for Aging

Research, a Washington-based nonprofit organization
on aging research

_____

How Does It Work? Vitamin C is a potent water-soluble
antioxidant that traps and disarms free radicals in the
watery part of tissues. It also regenerates exhausted vitamin E and all-important glutathione, and spurs enzymes
to search and destroy free radicals. Thus, for optimal
aging slowdown, it's critical that cells have enough of both
antioxidants E and C.

Together, vitamin C and vitamin E are the lions at the
gates—battling in different arenas, but in concert, against the
free radicals. Since your body does not store water-soluble
vitamin C, you must eat it regularly to keep cells supplied.

_____

Vitamin C has multiple complex effects on a variety of
biologic activities, perhaps more widespread than those
of any other nutrient. —National Cancer Institute, 1990

_____

What About Food? Vitamin C, unlike vitamin E, is plentiful in the food supply. So if you eat lots of vitamin C–rich
fruits and vegetables (at least five servings a day), you can
get fairly high doses of the vitamin, enough to discourage
certain chronic diseases, such as cataracts and cancer. But
to be safe, take a vitamin supplement in addition to, not
as a substitute for, fruits and vegetables. (Remember,
fruits and vegetables are packed with other antioxidants
essential to postponing aging.) Foods high in vitamin C
are sweet peppers, cantaloupe, pimientos, papaya, strawberries, Brussels sprouts, citrus fruits and juices, kiwi
fruit, broccoli, tomatoes and tomato juice.

Do You Need a Supplement? Yes, as insurance against the
increased demands of aging.

THE ANTIAGING PROMISE OF VITAMIN C

Here are fifteen ways vitamin C may fight aging and extend life, according to the latest research:

▲ Suppresses high blood pressure.
▲ Raises good-type HDL cholesterol.
▲ Reduces bad-type LDL cholesterol as well as Lp(a), another blood lipid hazard.
▲ Boosts levels of the body's most potent free radical enemy—glutathione.
▲ Inhibits bad-type LDL cholesterol from becoming toxic (rancid or oxidized) and able to clog arteries.
▲ Cleans fatty deposits from artery walls.
▲ Strengthens blood vessel walls, prevents bruising.
▲ Reduces the chances of heart-attack-inducing vascular spasms.
▲ Improves immune functioning.
▲ Cuts odds of asthma, chronic bronchitis and other lung and breathing problems.
▲ Prevents periodontal disease by fending off free radical attacks on gum tissue.
▲ Hinders oxidative damage to eyes, warding off cataracts and other age-related eye diseases.
▲ Protects sperm from free radical damage causing birth defects.
▲ Restores fertility in men.
▲ Fights cancer at least five ways: thwarts formation of carcinogens; blocks free radical DNA damage, a first step to cancer; prevents genes and viruses from switching on cancer activity; regulates immunity; slows tumor growth.

How Much? A daily 250 to 1,000 milligrams is considered adequate to combat the ordinary ravages of aging and age-related diseases, although many researchers take several thousand milligrams of vitamin C in the belief that higher doses convey additional antiaging benefits.

How Much Is Too Much? Vitamin C is very safe, although taking "too much" typically causes diarrhea, possibly nausea and heartburn in some persons. A "bowel tolerance" dose is highly individualistic and usually requires more than 1,000 milligrams a day, more if you are ill. No serious adverse effects were reported in eight recent studies from taking up to 10,000 milligrams of vitamin C daily for several years. There's no evidence vitamin C causes kidney stones. Nor do high doses of vitamin C cause "iron overload"—the harmful accumulation of iron in the body—in normal people, according to a review of research by Charles E. Butterworth, M.D., emeritus professor at the University of Alabama at Birmingham. Vitamin C supplements can exacerbate iron toxicity in those with genetic disorders in handling iron, notably a condition called hemochromatosis. Such persons should consult a physician before taking vitamin C supplements.

How Often? To keep your cells on total antioxidant alert with vitamin C, take your supplement quota three or four times a day rather than in one big dose. Throwing down a couple of 500-milligram pills at one time, particularly in the morning, instead of taking them throughout the day cheats your cells, because much of it is excreted in your urine. The body eliminates even large doses in twelve hours, and time-release doses in sixteen hours. The only way to keep levels of vitamin C continuously up in your blood is to take 500 milligrams every twelve hours, says

Alfred B. Ordman, biochemistry professor at Beloit College in Beloit, Wisconsin.

The evidence suggests that [by taking a few grams of vitamin C daily] one can add significant years to life and obvious life to years! —Dr. Emanuel Cheraskin, emeritus professor of medicine, University of Alabama. He takes 5,000 milligrams daily.

All-Around Antiaging Antioxidant

▲ ▲ ▲

(Why You Need Beta Carotene to Stop Aging)

Eat carrots, sweet potatoes, pumpkin, apricots and spinach to infuse cells with beta carotene. If you don't, be sure to take beta carotene pills. Even if you do eat lots of fruits and vegetables, it's still smart to take beta carotene as extra antiaging insurance.

To be sure, taking vitamin E and vitamin C can help save you from needless aging. But you still won't get maximum aging slowdown unless you also take in lots of beta carotene—from fruits and vegetables and/or pills. Beta carotene, the orange pigment first isolated from carrots a century and a half ago, has extra antioxidant powers that fill in where other vitamins and antioxidants leave off. Beta carotene appears plenty powerful at helping prevent and reverse cancer, heart disease, cataracts and failing immunity—in short, overall bodily deterioration.

Specifically, beta carotene protects the integrity of cells by snuffing out youth-stealing free radicals, primarily one known as singlet oxygen, that corrupt cells' genes, turn their fat rancid and toxic and destroy cell structure. Beta carotene also has additional antiaging powers. It can convert in the body to vitamin A, which has antiaging attributes of its own, especially in bolstering immunity.

How Beta Carotene Can Fight Aging

Blocks Cancer: One antioxidant you must not skimp on if you want to avoid cancer is beta carotene. More than one hundred studies show that people with high levels of beta carotene in their diet and in their blood are about half as likely to develop various cancers, notably of the lung, but also of the mouth, throat, esophagus, larynx, stomach, breast and bladder. A landmark Johns Hopkins University study found that people with low blood levels of beta carotene were four times more apt to develop a specific deadly type of lung cancer due to smoking.

Further, three Australian studies suggest that beta carotene blocks development of cancer of the cervix. Megadoses of beta carotene supplements reversed precancerous lesions of the mouth in 50 to 70 percent of subjects who took it. In men with colon cancer, doses of 30 milligrams of beta carotene a day inhibited specific cancer-promoting activity in cells by 44 percent after only two weeks and 57 percent after nine weeks. The activity remained low even six months after the men stopped taking the beta carotene. This suggests beta carotene is a cancer chemopreventive agent, says James Walter Kikendall, a gastroenterologist at Walter Reed Army Hospital Medical Center. A recent Australian study found that women with breast cancer who consumed the most beta carotene had twelve times better survival rates over a six-year period than those who ate the least. One explanation: Beta carotene blocks the proliferation of cancer cells.

Note: You can't expect beta carotene to save you quickly, especially from longtime cigarette smoking. It takes at least twelve years of high doses of beta carotene to thwart the onset of lung cancer, authorities say.

Prevents Heart Attacks: The evidence is compelling showing that beta carotene wards off cardiovascular disease, probably by keeping arteries from clogging. The most dramatic finding: A Harvard study showed that male physicians who took 50-milligram supplements of beta carotene every other day for six years had only half as many fatal heart attacks, strokes and heart disease incidents in general as doctors taking a dummy pill. Note: The protection kicked in only after two years, suggesting that beta carotene slows the progression of plaque buildup in arteries, says Charles Hennekens, M.D., director of the study.

In another Harvard study tracking ninety thousand female nurses, those eating the most beta carotene (more than 11,000 IU daily) had a 22 percent lower risk of heart disease than women getting less than 3,800 IU daily. The high–beta carotene eaters' risk of stroke was 37 percent lower. In a large-scale multicenter European study, those who took in the least beta carotene were at a 260 percent higher risk of a first heart attack than those who ate the most beta carotene.

Adults should take 10 milligrams (17,000 IU) to 30 milligrams (50,000 IU) of beta carotene daily for life!
—The Alliance for Aging Research, a Washington-based nonprofit organization on aging research

---

Prevents Strokes: Beta carotene seems to help prevent one of the most feared consequences of aging—stroke. Women who ate at least five beta carotene–rich carrots a week were 68 percent less likely to have a stroke compared with women who ate carrots once a month or less, according to a Harvard study of ninety thousand women. Eating lots of beta carotene–packed spinach also cut the stroke risk 40 percent.

Indeed, Harvard researcher Dr. JoAnn Manson says studies suggest that beta carotene has the strongest promise in preventing strokes, whereas vitamin E seems to work best against heart attacks.

High intakes of beta carotene may reduce cardio-vascular risk after two years. It takes at least twelve years for beta carotene to cut lung cancer risk, research indicates.

Stimulates Immune Functioning: Beta carotene supplements can greatly improve the makeup of your immune cells, according to tests at the University of Arizona. In a study of sixty older men and women (average age fifty-six), those who took 30 to 60 milligrams of beta carotene daily for two months had more natural killer cells, T-helper cells and activated lymphocytes. Such immune cells help protect the body from cancer and viral and bacterial infections, says study director Ronald R. Watson. Further, Dr. Simin Meydani at Tufts has found that Harvard physicians taking 50 milligrams of beta carotene every other day have significant rises of natural killer cells in their blood. Natural killer cells are particularly important in fighting off cancer.

What About Food? You can get lots of beta carotene in fruits and vegetables, although the beta carotene in supplements is better absorbed, according to tests at the U.S. Department of Agriculture. Your body can also absorb more beta carotene from vegetables, such as carrots, that are lightly cooked. Heavy cooking destroys beta carotene.

Do You Need a Supplement? If you want extra insurance against aging, many researchers favor a supplement of 10

FOODS WITH THE MOST ANTIAGING BETA CAROTENE

Food	Milligrams
Carrot juice: 1 cup	24.2
Sweet potato: 1 medium	10.0
Apricots, dried: 10 halves	6.2
Chicory, raw: 1 cup	6.2
Carrot, raw: 1 medium	5.7
Spinach, cooked: $1/2$ cup	4.9
Cantaloupe: $1/8$	4.0
Turnip greens, cooked: $1/2$ cup	3.9
Pumpkin, cooked: $1/2$ cup	3.7
Collard greens, cooked: $1/2$ cup	3.4
Swiss chard, cooked: $1/2$ cup	3.2
Kale, cooked: $1/2$ cup	3.0
Winter squash, cooked: $1/2$ cup	2.9
Apricots, fresh: 2	2.5
Spinach, raw: 1 cup	2.3
Tomato juice: 1 cup	2.2
Spaghetti squash, cooked: $1/2$ cup	1.9
Mustard greens, cooked: $1/2$ cup	1.9
Beet greens, cooked: $1/2$ cup	1.8
Grapefruit, pink or red: $1/2$	1.6
Mango: $1/2$	1.4
Dandelion greens, cooked: $1/2$ cup	1.4
Bell peppers, sweet red, raw: $1/2$ cup	1.1
Romaine lettuce, raw: 1 cup	1.1
Watermelon: 1 slice	1.1
Broccoli, cooked: $1/2$ cup	1.0

THE ANTIAGING PROMISE
OF BETA CAROTENE

▲ Prevents cancers of the lung, stomach and breast.
▲ Prevents strokes.
▲ Prevents heart attacks.
▲ Blocks oxidation of cholesterol that clogs arteries.
▲ Destroys tumor cells.
▲ Causes precancerous lesions in the mouth to disappear or regress.
▲ Stimulates immune functions.
▲ Prevents cataracts.

to 15 milligrams of beta carotene a day. Take it with meals because some fat in the diet is necessary for its absorption. Without a little fat, beta carotene pills are a waste. Also, a study at Massachusetts General Hospital in Boston found that taking divided doses of beta carotene three times a day with meals boosted blood concentrations of the vitamin three times higher than taking a single total dose once a day. Be sure the supplement label says beta carotene and not just vitamin A, which can be toxic.

How Much Is Too Much? Beta carotene is considered one of the most nontoxic of vitamins. Studies in Italy, for example, using 90 milligrams of beta carotene daily have shown no significant signs of toxicity. Hundreds of studies on laboratory animals using very high doses of beta carotene have detected virtually no toxicity. High doses, however, can cause yellowing of skin that disappears when you cut back on beta carotene.

Then in 1994 a study in Finland found that longtime heavy smokers who took 20 milligrams of beta carotene daily had an 18 percent greater risk of lung cancer than those not taking beta carotene. The finding was a shock to the scientific community, and most researchers do not believe it is valid for many scientifically complex reasons. Harvard researcher Julie Buring says: "The idea that the equivalent of seven or eight carrots a day causes cancer just doesn't make sense biologically."

Harvard investigator Dr. Charles Hennekens agrees: "The Finnish trial does not disprove the value of antioxidant vitamins, nor does it incriminate them as harmful."

In our heart of hearts we don't believe beta carotene is toxic. —Philip Taylor, chief of the National Cancer Institute's Division of Cancer Prevention Studies

---

In another study in China, National Cancer Institute researchers did find that taking 15 milligrams of beta carotene daily along with vitamin E and selenium reduced the incidence of lung cancer in smokers. However, the message seems clear: longtime heavy smokers cannot expect that taking beta carotene pills for a few years can erase the danger of lung cancer.

Some experts advise smokers not to take beta carotene supplements until more evidence is available, clarifying the Finnish finding.

Caution: Don't confuse beta carotene with plain retinol-type vitamin A, which is derived from animal foods, such as liver, and can build up to toxic levels in

your liver. Many multivitamin preparations contain high amounts of such retinol vitamin A. Adults should not take more than 5,000 to 10,000 IU of plain retinol vitamin A daily except on a physician's advice.

THE TRIPLE ANTIOXIDANT HIT

You can get antiaging help from any one of the three antioxidant staples, vitamin E, vitamin C and beta carotene. Each individually packs plenty of antioxidant power at fighting off bodily deterioration due to free radicals. But the three together are even more impressive. For example, here's what Harvard researchers found in epidemiological studies of eighty-seven thousand female nurses. In women getting lots of vitamin E, mostly from supplements (more than 200 IU daily), the odds of major cardiovascular disease dropped 34 percent. High intakes of beta carotene slashed heart disease risk 22 percent. High vitamin C intake reduced the odds 20 percent. But in women getting the highest amounts of all three antioxidants, heart disease risk dropped nearly 50 percent!

The same was true for strokes. High intake of all three antioxidants reduced the risk of strokes in the women by a startling 54 percent, far more than any of the vitamins alone. The probable reason: This cumulative antioxidant effect from all three is far better than any single antioxidant at retarding the steady clogging and deterioration of the arteries (atherosclerosis), thus preventing heart attacks and strokes.

For one thing, the three antioxidants work together to inhibit the oxidation of bad LDL cholesterol leading to plaque buildup in arteries. In a recent Australian study, researchers gave subjects daily doses of 900 milligrams of vitamin C, 200 milligrams of vitamin E and 18 milligrams of beta carotene. The result: The vitamins delayed the onset of oxidation of LDL cholesterol by 28 percent after three months. After six months, the antioxidation effect was even stronger.

Most remarkable, the three vitamins worked in sequence and in complementary fashion to delay LDL oxidation. When vitamin E was exhausted, beta carotene took over. However, if enough vitamin C was present, it regenerated vitamin E's powers. Thus the three antioxidants together seem most effective at reducing the danger of LDL oxidation.

The story seems much the same with cancer. Example: At Harvard's School of Dental Medicine, researchers have had great success in causing cancer to regress and disappear in hamsters by giving them vitamin E. However, they find that giving animals a mixture of vitamin E, beta carotene, vitamin C and the antioxidant glutathione is much more effective at making cancer vanish than is vitamin E alone.

All three vitamin staples of the antioxidant revolution—beta carotene, vitamin E and vitamin C—fight aging better than one or two alone.

Quick Fix for "Senility" and Other Aging Problems

▲ ▲ ▲

(Why You Need B Vitamins to Stop Aging)

It makes no sense not to take modest doses of B vitamins when the stakes are so high, the potential consequences of not doing it are so awful and the dangers of side effects are virtually nonexistent.

The astonishing antiaging news about the B vitamins is that they can help alleviate worry over your two most serious concerns as you grow old—your heart and your mental faculties. It's hard to separate the health impact of the many B vitamins. And if you lack one, you're likely to lack others. You need all of them to postpone aging, but three (vitamin B12, B6 and folic acid) are most critical because their antiaging powers are just now being discovered, thanks to dramatic new research. Yet millions of Americans live in needless jeopardy because they are unaware of the groundbreaking revelations about the powers of simple B vitamins to prevent and reverse some of the most dreaded consequences of aging.

THE ALARMING FACTS

▲ Vitamin B12 is probably the single most important nutrient affected by aging, says Dr. Robert Russell of Tufts.

▲ A startling 20 percent of people over age sixty-five were vitamin B12 deficient, according to a recent study.

▲ Sixty-seven percent of the cases of high homocysteine—an artery and brain toxin—among 1,160 elderly men and women was tied to low blood levels of one or more B vitamins.

How Vitamin B12 Can Fight Aging

Recovers Your Mind: Without vitamin B12 you can lose your mind. It can slowly be stolen away, often by a silent condition of aging that appears after middle age and leaves you depleted in vitamin B12, essential for proper mental functioning. You've probably never heard of this mind-robbing malady, although it's frighteningly widespread. According to one study by Robert Russell, an expert on the subject at the U.S. Department of Agriculture's Human Nutrition Research Center on Aging at Tufts University, it afflicts about 24 percent of people between ages sixty and sixty-nine; 32 percent between ages seventy and seventy-nine, and almost 40 percent after age eighty. Other studies suggest that fully 50 percent of all Americans after age sixty may suffer from this disorder. Yet nobody need get it or endure it because it is quickly prevented or counteracted by vitamin B12 supplements.

The condition is called atrophic gastritis, and it means that, as you get older, your stomach progressively secretes less hydrochloric acid, pepsin and intrinsic factor—a protein necessary to absorb vitamin B12 from food—than when you were younger. The consequence is a vitamin B12 deficiency that can be horrendous and usually quite unsuspected.

A vitamin B12 deficiency develops very slowly over many years and oddly, often affects the brain and nervous system entirely and nothing else. —Dr. John Lindenbaum, Columbia Presbyterian Medical Center

DON'T BE A VICTIM OF PSEUDO SENILITY

Commonly a B12 deficiency mimics "senility," dementia or Alzheimer's disease. Alarmingly, even mild B12 deficiencies, too subtle to show up in blood tests or to cause anemia, can result in neurological disorders, including dementia. Older people with blood B12 levels at the low end of the normal range have shown several neurologic symptoms including memory loss. Most improved when treated with B12. One major study revealed that fully 28 percent of patients with neurological disturbances with no signs of anemia attributable to B12 deficiency, still suffered dementia, loss of balance and other psychiatric disorders due to a lack of B12. Nor can you count on a blood test to detect vitamin B12 deficiency. Indeed, a recent study found that most of those with *normal* blood levels still lacked the B12 to adequately carry out metabolic functions.

The sooner a B12 deficiency is corrected, the better. Delaying as much as a year after neurological symptoms show up may be too late to totally stop or reverse the damage.

A B12 deficiency is a little like a growing cancer. It may start in midlife but not become dangerous until ten, twenty or thirty years later, when you are in your sixties or seventies, says Dr. John Lindenbaum, professor of medicine at Columbia Presbyterian Medical Center in New York City.

But why wait for a B12 deficiency to occur? Since it

has awful consequences and creeps up without warning, taking supplements of B12 is good insurance that can sharply cut your risk. In a recent study of four hundred older people, only 12 percent taking a daily supplement containing B12 (average 6 micrograms) had low B12 levels compared with a whopping 40 percent of non–vitamin takers. Non–vitamin takers were nearly three and a half times more apt to be deficient in B12.

Don't risk becoming a victim of pseudo senility. Take daily vitamin B12 pills as insurance, either alone or in a multiple-vitamin supplement.

Always suspect a vitamin B12 deficiency if an older person develops unexplained neuropsychiatric problems. —Dr. Robert Russell, Tufts University

------

What About Food? Only animal foods, such as meat, fish, chicken and dairy products have vitamin B12. This means vegetarians and people trying to avoid the perils of meat are even more susceptible than others to B12 deficiency.

Do You Need a B12 Supplement? Yes, as antiaging insurance, notably after age fifty. The reason pills can work when food doesn't: the crystalline forms of B12 put in supplements is absorbed even though stomach acid is low due to atrophic gastritis.

How Much? For some, a typical multiple-vitamin-mineral pill with 6 micrograms of B12 may fend off B12 deficiency. But there's no guarantee. Studies show that "a more appropriate dose for protection of older people is from 500 to 1,000 micrograms of B12 per day," says Dr. Lindenbaum. It takes that much to overcome severe malabsorption or advanced atrophic gastritis. When should you start taking it? Probably during your fifties or sixties. Deficiencies are quite unlikely before that age, says Dr. Lindenbaum.

How Much Is Too Much? "There is no toxicity to B12," says Dr. Russell. "It's harmless, so there is no danger in high doses, no overdose syndrome," agrees Dr. Lindenbaum. Single doses of 100,000 micrograms and long-term doses of 1,000 micrograms daily for five years have not caused toxic reactions, say experts. However, some allergic skin reactions have been reported.

> *Caution: A vitamin B12 deficiency can also cause pernicious anemia, a malabsorption of B12 usually due to an autoimmune disorder that blocks the stomach's production of intrinsic factor. The condition, which usually occurs after middle age, most frequently in women, requires medical attention and often requires lifelong injections of B12 or very high doses of B12 pills, given under a doctor's supervision.*

How Folic Acid Can Fight Aging

If your cells run low in folic acid, another monumentally important B vitamin in green leafy vegetables and legumes, you can kiss your youth goodbye. You are definitely on the rapid-aging track, as scientists have recently begun to discover. Folic acid, also called folate and folacin, is one of the brightest new superstars in antiaging research. And the vitamin has wide repercussions. Like B12, it can help save you from deteriorating mental functioning; it can help lift your mood, prevent and cure depression and turn off cancer. Even a marginal deficiency or "localized" deficiency within the cells of certain organs can make you more vulnerable to cancer. But folic acid's main claim to fame may be its ability to save you from a newly discovered villain that slowly mangles your arteries, triggering heart attacks and strokes.

Just taking a folic acid supplement of 400 to 1,000 micrograms a day could help save you from a heart attack, cancer and psychiatric disturbances. Don't take a chance of being deficient.

Unsuspected Heart Guardian: The right amount of folic acid in your blood can go a long way to squashing your vulnerability to cardiovascular disease. The reason: Elevated levels of a blood protein, homocysteine, are now considered a major risk factor for heart disease—as significant as or perhaps even more significant than cholesterol. High blood homocysteine triples your chances of heart disease. (For more on homocysteine hazards, see page 269.)

The three B vitamins, but particularly folic acid, spur enzymes to metabolize homocysteine, keeping it in check. If B vitamins are lacking, it soars to hazardous levels, leading to blocked arteries. According to a 1995 Tufts study of 1,041 men and women, ages sixty-seven to ninety-six, those with the highest homocysteine were twice as apt to have narrowed neck arteries determined by ultrasound as those with the least homocysteine. Amazing, but true: Benign doses of B vitamins rapidly whisk homocysteine right out of your system.

The vitamins deliver a kind of one, two, three punch against homocysteine. Of the three, folic acid is most powerful, followed by B6 and B12. According to Tufts research, if you get less than 350 micrograms of folic acid daily, you are apt to have high homocysteine. One study of elderly people found that those getting little folic acid (200 micrograms daily) were six times more likely to have dangerously high homocysteine than those getting more folic acid (400 micrograms daily).

THE ALARMING FACTS

▲ The average American over age fifty is woefully deficient in folic acid—taking in a mere 235 micrograms of folic acid daily—far too little to curb homocysteine or prevent cervical cancer.
▲ The less folic acid in your blood, the more your arteries are apt to be narrowed and clogged, according to Tufts research.
▲ Smokers need three times more folic acid (at least 600 micrograms daily) to achieve the same blood levels as nonsmokers.

Cancer Turn-Off: Folic acid can actually help block and reverse cancer, even after premalignant cells are evident. Target cells, for example in the lung or cervix, can develop a "localized" deficiency of folic acid, not common to the whole body and undetectable by ordinary blood tests. This makes you vulnerable to cancer takeover in the deficient tissues.

In striking studies at the University of Alabama, women infected with the HP virus, a common culprit in cervical cancers, who had low folic acid in red blood cells of the cervix were five times more likely to develop precancerous changes leading to cancer than those with higher folic acid. Without folic acid, chromosomes are more apt to break at "fragile" points, says Charles Butterworth, Jr., M.D., University of Alabama at Birmingham. This allows the virus to slip into the healthy cell's genetic material, promoting DNA damage that precedes cancer.

Other studies show that a lack of folic acid makes you more susceptible to lung, esophageal and breast cancer and polyps that precede colon cancer.

Folic acid may also save you from colon cancer, especially before age sixty. In a study of about sixteen thousand women and ninety-five hundred men, Harvard researchers found that those getting the most folic acid had the lowest incidence of polyps (precancerous growths) in the colon. Women who ate about 700 micrograms of folic acid daily had only two-thirds the risk of polyps as women consuming 166 micrograms. Those who took supplements fared best. The theory: Folic acid helps block a process that activates cancer genes.

Mind Savior: Folic acid can help preserve your mental faculties as you grow older. Psychiatric symptoms, including memory loss, depression and dementia, are much more common in people, especially the elderly, who have low levels of folic acid, according to a many studies, says Dr. E. H. Reynolds of King's College School of Medicine and Dentistry in London. He cites one study in which elderly patients with mental disorders, especially dementia, were three times more apt to have low folic acid than others their age. Even healthy people with low folic acid intake scored lower on abstract thinking ability and memory. Depression has been relieved by as little as 400 micrograms daily of folic acid in those with a deficiency.

The young suffer too. In one German study at the University of Giessen, a lack of folic acid in the diets of young men signified poor emotional stability, poor concentration, more introversion and lack of self-confidence. All these conditions improved dramatically when they got adequate folic acid for eight weeks. Moderate doses as found in multivitamin pills did the trick.

ANTIAGING SECRETS OF THE EXPERTS
Rene Malinow, M.D.:
Called the Father of Homocysteine Research
Professor of Medicine at
Oregon Health Sciences University

To keep homocysteine normal, Dr. Malinow takes a separate supplement of 1,000 micrograms (1 milligram) of folic acid plus 400 micrograms in a multiple-vitamin pill for a total of 1.4 milligrams of folic acid daily.

"Folic acid is cheap and innocuous and it usually reduces homocysteine to normal in a few days," says Dr. Malinow.

One reason for folic acid's brain effects may be its ability to help break down homocysteine, which is a known neurotoxin, causing brain cells to self-destruct.

How Much? Four hundred micrograms of folic acid a day may suppress homocysteine hazards and cancer threats, and even correct deficiencies leading to psychiatric disorders. You can usually find that dose in a multivitamin pill and in your diet. But to be on the ultra safe side, especially if you already have high homocysteine or heart disease, some experts advise 1,000 to 5,000 microgram supplements of folic acid daily to control homocysteine. In one study, a high folic acid diet did not normalize homocysteine in most subjects.

What About Food? Foods such as dried beans, spinach, collard greens and citrus fruits contain fairly high doses of folic acid. However, your body generally can absorb and use at most 50 percent of the folic acid in food, so although eating high folic-acid foods fights aging, it is not as reliable in reducing homocysteine as taking supplements.

How Much Is Too Much? Doses of 5,000 to 10,000 micrograms of folic acid daily have not caused noticeable side effects. Very high doses of folic acid could mask symptoms of B12 deficiency and pernicious anemia, unless proper diagnostic tests are used. If you have any reason to suspect you might have this condition, check it out before taking over 1,000 micrograms of folic acid a day.

Caution: If you use antibiotics for prolonged periods or frequently take antacids at mealtime, your ability to absorb folic acid drops significantly—no matter how old you are.

How Vitamin B6 Can Fight Aging

If you don't get enough vitamin B6, you may be more vulnerable to the classic signs of aging—mainly a failing immune system, declining mental status, compromised heart health, various infectious diseases and possibly cancer, according to Tufts University researchers. For example, a vitamin B6 deficiency leads to reduced production of T-cells, T-helper cells and antibodies, all disease-fighting substances of the immune system. Worse yet, older people require about 20 percent more B6 than younger people. After age forty you start running low on B6, mainly because you absorb it less efficiently.

Surprisingly, a lack of vitamin B6 is widespread. Amer-

THE VANISHING CANCERS

People who puff twenty to thirty cigarettes a day are apt to have precancerous cells in mucus or phlegm they cough up. And such precancerous cells can become malignant, triggering full-blown lung cancer. But if you could eliminate the precancerous cells, the threat of lung cancer would diminish. That's what happened when researchers at the University of Alabama gave smokers very high daily doses of folic acid (10,000 micrograms) and vitamin B12 (1,000 micrograms). Amazingly, large numbers of the premalignant cells just disappeared within four months, even though subjects continued to smoke.

Researchers believe such precancerous cell changes occur because of a "localized" deficiency of folic acid and B12 within lung tissue. When the tissue is suffused with the B vitamins, the precancerous cells become normal again. This does not mean, they caution, that taking vitamins or correcting a vitamin deficiency is a substitute for stopping smoking. However, the study does illustrate the formidable cancer preventive power of vitamins and what happens when you lack them.

icans typically take in 50 to 75 percent less vitamin B6 than the recommended dietary allowances (RDA). Older people are worse off partly because they lose some ability to use B vitamins. About one-third of the elderly have marginal vitamin B6 levels, according to Tufts research.

Boosts Immune Functioning: Being low in B6 decimates the warriors of your immune system; the percentage of lymphocytes goes down significantly; the production of interleukin-2, the stuff that encourages all-important T-cell growth, diminishes. But researchers at Tufts have completely restored such functioning to normal in older people by giving them daily supplements of B6 for three weeks. The effective dose: 1.9 milligrams a day for women and 2.88 milligrams for men. Extra large doses—50 milligrams per day—did not rejuvenate immune functioning further, say researchers.

Saves Blood Vessels: B6 is a big player in the battle against homocysteine, the newly discovered destroyer of blood vessels. B6 is the second line of defense. Folic acid affects one enzyme that breaks down homocysteine. But B6 is needed to work on a separate enzyme that also breaks down homocysteine. Studies consistently reveal that without enough B6 in your blood, homocysteine can build up, damaging arteries and provoking heart attacks and strokes. There's some evidence B6 also hinders dangerous blood clotting.

Improves Brain Functioning: In one Dutch study, 20 milligrams a day of B6 taken for three months improved the long-term memories of men in their seventies. The researchers speculated that adequate vitamin B6 may retard age-related memory decline.

How Much? Typical multivitamin pills contain 3 milligrams of B6, which is enough to correct deficiencies and boost immunity. Supplements of 10 to 50 milligrams of B6 a day may be needed to reduce homocysteine, studies show.

What About Food? Foods rich in B6 are seafood, whole grains, nuts, soybeans, bananas, sweet potatoes and prunes.

How Much Is Too Much? It's safest to stick to a dose of no more than 50 milligrams of B6 daily. Avoid doses of more than 200 milligrams a day. High doses, especially over the long term, can cause neurological symptoms. Doses of 500 to 1,000 milligrams daily have produced nervous system toxicity.

A Passport to More
Energy, Longer Life

▲　▲　▲

(Why You Need Chromium to Stop Aging)

If you're age twenty or older, chances are nearly
100 percent you lack chromium and are thus aging
much faster than you need to. Take a daily chromium tablet of 200 micrograms to help stop it.

Picture this: The rats just kept living, roaming their laboratory cages, oblivious to the fact that they should have
expired long ago of old age. Ordinarily, rats live two and a
half years. But another winter, spring, summer and fall
passed, and nearly all were still alive. On average they
lived a full year longer than normal, exceeding their usual
life span by an astonishing one-third. (In humans that
would mean stretching the average life span from 75 years
to about 102.)

Their longevity secret? They had been eating modest
doses of chromium picolinate, a particular form of the
vital trace mineral chromium that's found in low doses in
certain foods. "I wasn't surprised," says Gary Evans, Ph.D.,
a professor of chemistry in the Minnesota State University
system at Bemidji, Minnesota, and a prominent chromium
researcher. "I expected them to live longer because they
had many of the characteristics of lab animals on
restricted calorie diets, and those animals always live
longer," he says.

In short, chromium picolinate induced some desirable bodily changes—such as a decrease in insulin and blood sugar—just as restricting calories does, but without an actual cutback in food.

Sound promising? You bet. Who wouldn't prefer a life-extending pill to dieting? There's no proof, of course, that the rat experience will translate into equal gains in human longevity. But there is boundless evidence that chromium does help control insulin and blood sugar, and this achievement, many experts think, is a ticket to a longer, more vigorous life.

THE ALARMING FACTS

- At least 90 percent of Americans have a serious chromium shortage, typically taking in less than half of what experts say is the bare minimum of 50 micrograms a day.
- It's virtually impossible to get enough chromium from food. You have to eat 3,000 to 4,000 calories a day to get even 50 micrograms. To get the recommended 200 micrograms, you must eat more than 12,000 calories a day, say Department of Agriculture experts.
- Without enough chromium, excesses of insulin and glucose (sugar) can build up in your blood, exposing you to diabetes, heart disease and other symptoms of premature aging.
- One in four Americans—fifty million adults—may unknowingly suffer from mild to severe blood glucose intolerance, also called carbohydrate sensitivity. Forty million of them could benefit from taking chromium. You could be one of them.

WHY YOU ABSOLUTELY CAN'T AGE SLOWLY WITHOUT CHROMIUM

The single overriding reason to take chromium is to save yourself from accelerated aging brought on by too much of the hormone insulin in your blood. It's an insidious, largely undetected disorder that comes with age, and it can push you into diabetes at the same time it destroys your arteries. Authorities increasingly blame an excess of insulin for polluting our bloodstreams with dangerous amounts of blood sugar, bad-type LDL cholesterol and triglycerides, and for directly stimulating heart disease, diabetes and possibly cancer. One-fourth of Americans past middle age have a serious insulin disorder, yet few suspect it or know how harmful it can be, because it produces few symptoms until the damage is done. Medically, it has been labeled "insulin resistance—the secret killer."

I call chromium the "geriatric nutrient," because everybody starts to really need it past age thirty-five.
—Dr. Gary Evans, Bemidji State University in Minnesota

Essentially, it means your cells are less efficient at using insulin to process blood sugar than when you were younger. Cells become less sensitive or "resistant" to insulin. In efforts to control blood sugar, your body may then dump more insulin in your blood. If the insulin is too weak, your blood sugar also can soar. In any event, your blood is awash with abnormally high loads of useless dysfunctional insulin and sugar that conspire to destroy your arteries by stimulating processes that build up plaque, leading to heart attacks and strokes. Blood insulin and sugar overloads can also push you into irreversible full-fledged diabetes in mid to late life. Many experts consider excessive insulin a major instigator of a constellation of hazards responsible for our massive heart disease and diabetes toll. (For more details on insulin's potential damage, see page 281.)

Now, the amazing news: Your insulin (and blood sugar) levels soar and wreak havoc if you lack chromium. Indeed, a chromium deficiency begets insulin resistance. And taking chromium supplements can help cure and prevent this dreadful insulin imbalance. Essentially, chromium revs up insulin action, so you need less to do the job. Fully 80 percent of the controlled studies found that taking chromium improved insulin efficiency or improved blood cholesterol and triglycerides, according to a recent review by Walter Mertz, Ph.D., a pioneering chromium researcher formerly at the U.S. Department of Agriculture. It's unclear exactly how chromium works, but in test-tube experiments, it attaches tightly to insulin, enhancing by up to one hundred times the hormone's main mission of converting glucose into carbon dioxide.

Thus, taking chromium can help save you from the ravages of rapid aging by optimizing insulin activity.

Everybody needs at least 200 micrograms of chromium a day. Taking chromium can help save you from heart disease, diabetes and possibly cancer. —Dr. Richard A. Anderson, U.S. Department of Agriculture

---

The Sweet Chromium Robbers

If you eat sugary foods, you need chromium even more. Sugar can destroy what little dietary chromium you take in. So your body is hit with a double whammy—high sugar and even less chromium—that conspire to spike blood insulin and sugar, accelerating aging. Either table sugar or high fructose corn syrup (in soft drinks and other processed foods), and notably both together, wash chromium right out of the body, worsening borderline deficiencies. Eating a third of your calories in sugar causes three times the losses in chromium as eating 10 percent of calories in sugar.

HIDDEN PRO-AGING TIME BOMB

Most alarming is the fact that the ill effects of a chromium deficiency are generally mistaken for "normal aging." The decline is gradual and subtle. "It usually takes years for signs of chromium deficiency to show up," says Dr. Richard Anderson. "Chromium levels just gradually go down, and after decades, your cholesterol is going up, your insulin is going up, your HDLs are going down and your glucose is going up—and you're in trouble. Most people think these things just happen because you get older. Actually, they happen because of a diet with too little chromium and too much sugar. And they are preventable."

Take chromium to ensure against the monstrous and hidden dangers of excessive blood insulin and sugar that otherwise can creep up with age, destroying your health and shortening your life. Chromium helps normalize blood sugar and insulin before they do irreparable damage. Chromium is not a quick fix for everyone, but it is a very inexpensive antiaging insurance policy for virtually all of us.

How Chromium Can Fight Aging

Controls Hazardous Insulin: Chromium increases the power of insulin to process sugar, so you need less insulin to do the job, and blood levels drop. If chromium is low, you need about ten times more insulin to process sugar, says Dr. Anderson. Thus, with adequate chromium, much less insulin circulates in the blood to attack artery walls, precipitating atherosclerosis, and possibly plunging you into adult-onset (Type II) diabetes. By reactivating insulin, chromium alleviates some of the danger of "insulin resistance" that comes on with age. Chromium can even improve insulin resistance in diabetics, according to several studies. A daily 200 micrograms of chromium picolinate improved insulin resistance in 62 percent of women with Type II diabetes and 50 percent of men with the disorder within ten days, according to Israeli research.

If you take people in the general population with slightly elevated blood sugar and give them chromium supplements, you'll see a drop in blood sugar in 80 to 90 percent of them. —Dr. Richard A. Anderson, U.S. Department of Agriculture

---

Normalizes Blood Sugar: Excessive blood sugar promotes diabetes and all the destruction that goes with it. Studies show that if you have high blood sugar, chromium supplements will bring it down. Amazingly, if you have low blood sugar, chromium will bring it up. Chromium has an "adaptogen" effect, says Dr. Anderson, meaning it normalizes blood sugar, no matter what the imbalance. This probably results from chromium's ability to normalize insulin, he says. In one double-blind study of eleven diabetics, taking chromium caused fasting blood sugar to fall

24 percent in eight of them, presumably those deficient in chromium.

If your blood sugar is normal, chromium has no effect on it.

Lowers Blood Cholesterol: A decade of studies shows that chromium lowers bad-type LDL cholesterol and raises good-type HDL cholesterol. One recent study found that giving twenty-three men 200 micrograms of chromium boosted artery-cleansing HDL levels 11 percent. Blood insulin levels also dropped in those with high levels to begin with. Another eight-week study at Auburn University in Alabama found that men with low cholesterol who received 200 micrograms of niacin-bound chromium (ChromeMate brand) showed an average drop of 14 percent in total cholesterol. Chromium—250 micrograms a day—also pushed up HDLs in elderly heart disease patients by about 20 percent, Israeli investigators found.

Boosts Immune Functioning: By making insulin more efficient, chromium improves immune functions. Insulin helps direct many immune functions, such as stimulating interferon and T-lymphocytes—white cells that destroy germs.

Prevents Heart Disease: Three decades ago, investigators noted that people dying of heart disease had remarkably low concentrations of chromium in their aortas. In more recent studies, researchers have found that heart patients have up to 40 percent lower blood levels of chromium than healthy individuals. Further, animals deprived of chromium suffer extensive plaque buildup in their arteries. Injecting animals with chromium has caused plaque in their aortas to shrink, reversing atherosclerosis.

Many experts insist that insulin and blood sugar disorders, partly correctable by chromium, are far more important factors in heart disease than high blood cholesterol.

Boosts Antiaging Hormone: Chromium may also curb signs of aging by promoting rises in the all-important antiaging hormone, DHEA (dehydroepiandrosterone). High insulin levels squash production of DHEA by inhibiting an enzyme that converts a chemical into DHEA. Chromium picolinate supplements boost DHEA production. In one test of postmenopausal women by Dr. Evans, levels of DHEA dropped about 10 percent after they stopped taking 200 micrograms of chromium daily for four to six months.

DHEA is a hormone that dwindles dramatically as you age, along with declining insulin efficiency. At age seventy-five you have only 10 percent as much DHEA as you had at age twenty-five, according to prominent French researcher Etienne-Emile Baulieu of the College de France. In tests, he is giving elderly people low doses of synthetic DHEA as an antiaging agent. Evidence indicates DHEA may improve brain function, memory loss, immunity, muscle fatigue and bone fragility and perhaps may help block cancer.

What About Food? Don't depend on food for antiaging chromium; it is an unreliable source. U.S. Department of Agriculture scientists recently designed the best diets they could think of; yet the most chromium in the "super diets" was still a mere 24 micrograms per 1,000 calories. Foods high in chromium are brewer's yeast, broccoli, barley, liver, lobster tail, shrimp, whole grains, mushrooms and some brands of beer, due to contamination during processing. However, much chromium in food is not well absorbed.

THE ANTIAGING PROMISE OF CHROMIUM

Taking chromium supplements may help:

▲ Lower insulin levels.
▲ Lower triglycerides.
▲ Raise good-type HDL cholesterol.
▲ Discourage artery-clogging and heart disease.
▲ Lower bad-type blood cholesterol.
▲ Normalize blood sugar.
▲ Reduce your risk of adult-onset diabetes.
▲ Thwart cancer growth.
▲ Boost immune functioning.
▲ Increase energy.
▲ Increase lean body mass.
▲ Rev up production of antiaging hormone DHEA.
▲ Extend life.

What Type of Supplement? Choose organic, "biologically active" forms of chromium. That includes the popular chromium picolinate—a particular organic-type supplement, developed at the U.S. Department of Agriculture. It is reputedly readily absorbed and used by the body and has been widely and successfully tested in both animal and humans. Also good are the niacin-bound chromiums, such as ChromeMate and Solgar GTF chromium. Chromium chloride, often put in multiple-vitamin-mineral pills, is less effective. It is inorganic, which means your body must convert it to an active type before it does any good; some people don't do this well. But any type of chromium is better than none, say authorities.

How Much? To prevent chronic diseases as you age, ordinary healthy teenagers and adults need about 200 micrograms of chromium a day. Chromium expert Dr. Evans advises 400 micrograms for men. If you are diabetic or trying to improve blood cholesterol or triglycerides, you need more—from 400 to 1,000 micrograms daily, say authorities.

If you can find 200 micrograms of the right type of chromium, such as chromium picolinate, in a multivitamin pill, go for it. But such multi pills rarely include enough of the right type of organic chromium. Usually you must take an individual chromium supplement of 200 micrograms.

Who Should Take Chromium? If everyone took chromium, starting in their teens—at least before age twenty—much premature aging could be averted, along with heart disease and diabetes in midlife and old age, says USDA scientist Dr. Richard Anderson. Chromium levels decline with each decade of life. However, it's never too late. At any age, you may arrest the progression toward heart disease and diabetes by starting to take chromium.

> *Caution: If you are diabetic, take chromium supplements only with a doctor's supervision, because the mineral may alter insulin requirements.*

How Fast Does It Work? Improvements in insulin and blood sugar are fast—within a few days to a few weeks. It takes a few weeks to a couple of months—depending on the dose—to see improvements in blood cholesterol and triglycerides, says Dr. Anderson.

Can You Be Tested for Chromium Deficiency? At present there is no reliable test for chromium deficiency.

How Much Is Too Much? Chromium toxicity is very low. Agriculture's Dr. Anderson says you could take three hundred times the recommended dose of 200 micrograms without "getting in trouble." But since chromium might be deposited in the liver and kidneys and since extra high doses are generally unnecessary, there's no reason for most people to go above 200 micrograms per day in a supplement as general antiaging protection.

See Your Immune System Grow Young Again

▲ ▲ ▲

(Why You Need Zinc to Stop Aging)

Don't let your immune system fall asleep, plunging you into premature aging, just because you lack a little zinc. Even mild deficiencies, undetected by blood tests, put you in needless jeopardy. And don't think it can't happen to you. "I was shocked to discover my own cells were low in zinc," says leading zinc researcher Dr. Ananda Prasad, who now takes 15 to 20 milligrams of zinc daily.

Tucked in the neck behind the top of the breastbone of every human being is a small pouch, called the thymus gland—a maestro of wizardry that orchestrates the workings of the immune system throughout your entire life. Unfortunately, as you age, the thymus gland, big and robust in youth (at birth, it's bigger than your heart) shrivels up, losing its power. The progressive shrinking starts soon after puberty, and by age sixty, the thymus gland is usually a mere shadow of its early self, reflecting a rapid decline in immune functioning. This shrinkage of the thymus is one of the most spectacular signs of aging. By age forty, "you can't find the thymus on an X ray," says Dr. William Adler, an immunologist at the National Institute on Aging.

The situation becomes grim. Without an active thymus gland, the immune system's T-cells do not mature enough to spot foreign invaders, so you are more prone to infections. Without the direction of T-cells, B-cells falter in their ability to make antibodies. Fact: The death rate from influenza at age seventy is thirty-five times higher than at age ten, says Dr. Adler.

Until very recently, experts considered the slow decline of the thymus gland an irreversible condition of advancing age, accounting for much of the deteriorating immunity that comes with age and dooms us to infections, cancer and autoimmune diseases in our later years.

But it's simply not true. Exciting experiments now show that the saga of the aging, shrinking thymus gland is mostly myth; it's decline is stoppable and reversible, its youthful powers retrievable. Indeed, it can be rejuvenated even late in life by the remarkable authority of a mineral called zinc.

THE ALARMING FACTS

▲ One in three healthy Americans over age fifty has a zinc deficiency and rarely suspects it.
▲ More than 90 percent of older healthy Americans do not take in the RDA (recommended dietary allowance) for zinc.
▲ You have to take in about 2,400 calories a day to get the RDA for zinc.
▲ Countless millions of Americans have depressed immunity due to needless and reversible mild deficiencies of zinc.

HOW ZINC FIGHTS AGING BY REJUVENATING IMMUNITY

Famous Mice Experiments: In pioneering experiments on aged mice, Dr. Nicola Fabris, at the Italian National Center on Aging in Ancona, found that daily low doses of zinc produced an astonishing 80 percent restoration of thymus gland

ZINC GOES ZIP IN MIDDLE AGE

You're apt to be low in antiaging zinc if:

▲ You don't eat at least 2,400 calories a day.
▲ You're a vegetarian. Zinc is mostly in meat, seafood and poultry.
▲ You have cut back on meat.
▲ You eat lots of fiber. Fiber blocks zinc absorption.
▲ You are on a calorie-fat reducing diet.
▲ You are past age fifty. Your ability to absorb zinc flags.

function. With it came a rejuvenation of immune functioning. The thymus gland, for example, secretes thymulin, an all-important hormone that stimulates production of T-cells. Infused with zinc, the old mice's thymus glands began churning out more biologically active thymulin and T-cells. "Zinc causes the hibernating thymus to come alive again," says Dr. Fabris. The thymus doesn't really disappear with age; it simply appears to shrink because it becomes inactive, he says. By replenishing missing zinc, we can turn back the immune clock, restoring thymus efficiency to what it was at a much younger age. In the elderly, that means reclaiming an immune system typical of their forties, he insists.

Needless Tragedy: Absolutely true, agrees Ananda S. Prasad, M.D., professor of medicine at Wayne State University School of Medicine and an authority on zinc. In fact, he sees the failure to recognize zinc's antiaging powers as a needless human tragedy of monumental and growing proportions. Dr. Prasad's research reveals that about one in three seemingly healthy Americans over age fifty has a mild zinc deficiency, not detectable in typical blood tests. Thus more than twenty million Americans are unknowingly at high risk of infections and the degenerative diseases of aging. It's a situation Dr. Prasad calls "appalling," especially since it is so easily fixable.

Revives Immune Functions: Astonishingly, Dr. Prasad has also demonstrated that a dime's worth of zinc a day may prevent a fortune in health care and suffering. Mildly zinc-deficient subjects, ages fifty to eighty, who took 30 milligrams of zinc gluconate every day for six months, saw their immune functioning come dramatically alive. Their output and activity of thymulin, the hormone that is critical to the formation of lymphocytes, jumped by more than 40 percent. Also, the thymus gland's production of interleukin 1, which is a very important substance in boosting T-cell production, nearly doubled. It's proof positive that deteriorating immunity due to a failing thymus gland is not ordained by aging but by a zinc deficiency that can be reversed.

I'm confident that zinc is an antiaging agent. —Dr. Nicola Fabris, Italian National Center on Aging, an authority on zinc

-----

It's Never Too Late to Prolong Life: French researchers also recently found that even the immune systems of the very old can be salvaged. They gave a group of institutionalized people, 73 to 106 years old, 20 milligrams of zinc a day. Their thymulin activity shot up as much as 50 percent within a couple of months. Almost all the subjects were deficient in zinc to begin with. There were no side effects. Especially fascinating, researchers noted, zinc also markedly pushed up blood levels of albumin, a protein notoriously

ANTIAGING SECRETS OF THE EXPERTS

William A. Pryor, Ph.D.
Director of the Biodynamics Institute,
Louisiana State University

Dr. Pryor has studied free radicals and antioxidants for nearly thirty years and is a leading authority in the field.

Here's what Dr. Pryor takes every day to forestall free radical damage and aging:

▲ Vitamin E (natural form)—400 IU.
▲ Vitamin C—500 milligrams.
▲ Beta carotene—15 milligrams.
▲ Multivitamin-mineral tablet with zinc and selenium.

"I also like coenzyme Q-10 and take it sometimes.

"I've been taking vitamin supplements for about twenty years and I'm sorry I didn't eat better and start taking vitamins at around age ten."

low in most elderly. Albumin is a biomarker of longevity—those with high levels live longer. Thus zinc indirectly may extend life.

Zinc also stimulates production of gamma interferon, a substance essential to proper immune functioning. Interferon production drops in aging humans and mice.

In mice cells, Dr. Fabris and colleagues completely restored interferon production lost to aging by administering zinc.

Fights Free Radicals: Zinc provides global protection against aging by functioning as an antioxidant. If you are low in zinc, destructive free radicals roam your body, attacking cells and promoting general breakdown and aging. Studies find that zinc-deficient animals have 15 to 20 percent higher levels of rampaging free radicals than animals with normal zinc. There's evidence that a lack of zinc permits excessive free radical activity incriminated in age-related macular degeneration (vision robber), infertility, cancer and forms of degenerative brain disease.

How Much? A daily dose of 15 to 30 milligrams of zinc is usually enough to preserve immune functioning as you age or to reverse deficiencies, revitalizing the thymus gland and restoring youthful immune activity. However, some people over age seventy-five may need doses of 50 milligrams or more of zinc daily to substantially retrieve thymus activity, says Dr. Fabris. Such high doses, especially in the elderly, should not be taken without careful medical supervision, for high doses of zinc can depress immunity.

What Type? Zinc gluconate is preferable, says Dr. Prasad, because it is less irritating to the GI tract than the common zinc sulfate found in supplements. Also, common zinc sulfate and zinc oxide are poorly absorbed and used by the body. Better absorbed are the chelated forms—zinc citrate, zinc gluconate and the newest, zinc monomethionine. You can sometimes get enough zinc in a multivitamin-mineral pill to deter aging. Some tablets contain 15 milligrams of zinc. But check to be sure it is in an easily absorbed form, such as zinc gluconate or citrate.

What About Food? It's difficult to get enough zinc in the diet, especially for vegetarians and people who are cutting down on meat. Highest in zinc is seafood, notably shellfish and especially oysters, the richest source known. (Always cook them or eat canned oysters.) Lean meats are also a rich source. Cereals, nuts and seeds are relatively high in zinc, but they also contain agents that reduce zinc absorption.

How Much Is Too Much? Some experts fear that high doses of zinc interfere with other nutrients and can lower immunity. Since it only takes 15 to 30 milligrams daily to correct deficiencies and boost immunity in most people, there is no reason to take higher doses. In any event, don't take more than 50 milligrams daily except on a doctor's advice. At that dose or under, "we have not seen any adverse effects," says Dr. Prasad.

Can You Tell If You Are Zinc Deficient? You cannot depend on a simple blood test to detect zinc deficiency. What's needed is an assessment of the amount of zinc in the white blood cells, which is an easy test in a doctor's office, says Dr. Prasad. But chances are if you're in midlife you are at least marginally deficient in zinc and you are aging too fast as a result. Since modest zinc doses usually correct a deficiency and are not harmful, it makes sense to take them as a precaution as you get older.

The Antiaging Mineral
You Must Take

▲ ▲ ▲

(Why You Need Calcium to Stop Aging)

Why play Russian roulette with your youth when calcium can erase so many aging fears? It's smart to start getting lots of calcium now whether you are age eight or age eighty.

Your Stone Age ancestors ate lots of calcium. And you don't. That's one reason your bones grow fragile and break, your endocrine system gets screwed up and your cell growth regulation can run amok as you get older. In short, one more reason you may collapse into old age. Yes, calcium is much more than a bone savior. Your cells need calcium to function properly. Our bodies were designed by evolution and genetics to run on extraordinarily high amounts of calcium compared with the paltry amounts we get today. Our Stone Age ancestors ate 2,000 to 3,000 milligrams a day of calcium, mostly by foraging for wild plants. That's five times more than today's average—a mere 500 milligrams for women ages thirty-five to seventy-four, according to a large-scale government study. Moreover, the hazard worsens with age, as you tend to absorb less calcium with the passing years.

AMAZING ANTIAGING CALCIUM STORY

It surprised even the most passionate advocates of calcium and was declared one of the ten most important medical developments of 1993 by the *Harvard Health Letter*. A study by French scientists at INSERM, the government's main medical research agency, found that taking calcium pills plus vitamin D for only a year and a half dramatically suppressed bone fractures in women over age eighty! In the study, 3,270 healthy women over age eighty took a daily 1,200 milligrams of elemental calcium plus 800 IU of vitamin D3 (cholecalciferol) or a placebo (inactive pill).

During the study's eighteen months, the supplement takers had an astonishing 43 percent fewer hip fractures and 32 percent fewer fractures of the wrist, arm and pelvis than the nonsupplemented women. This proves beyond a doubt the incredible power of such supplements to spare suffering and prolong life. Hip fractures leave many irreversibly unable to walk, and about 20 percent don't survive.

But there's no need to let this dreary situation drag you into premature old age. You can stop some of the damage from too little calcium, no matter how old you are. Truth is, it's better to get calcium at an early age, but it's never too late. To fend off aging, start now. Calcium has performed miracles for many in their eighties.

THE ALARMING FACTS

▲ Most Americans get only half the calcium they need to postpone aging.

▲ Calcium deficiency is not just a female problem.
Men, too, needlessly suffer chronic diseases
because they lack calcium.

▲ Less than half of American children get the recommended dietary allowances for calcium.

HOW CALCIUM CAN FIGHT AGING

Keeps Bones Young: To prevent brittle bones and old-age
skeletal deformities, you need calcium at every age,
according to impressive research. The idea is to maximize
bone mass early in life and minimize bone thinning in
later life. You have your thickest, strongest bones between
ages twenty and thirty, and most of the buildup happens
during adolescence.

That's why it's critical for the young, especially girls, to
load up on calcium before puberty, if possible, and certainly before age twenty-five. For example, women with the
strongest bones in middle and old age drank the most milk
before age twenty-five, according to a recent British study.
Steven A. Abrams at Children's Nutrition Research Center
in Houston says girls need the most calcium during bone-
forming activity that occurs just before and after the start
of puberty (average age ten in girls), so it's smart to
increase calcium intake several years before that, he urges.

However, if you missed calcium when young, don't
despair. Getting it later can intervene to help prevent
bone loss in the spine, hip and wrist well after
menopause, and even into very old age. Fully twenty-
seven studies published since 1988 show the benefits of
calcium in building bone mass and preventing bone loss
or bone fragility, according to leading expert Robert P.
Heaney, M.D., John A. Creighton University Professor at
Creighton University.

Reducing hip fractures by 20 percent would save about $2 billion a year in health care costs. —Dr. Robert Heaney, Creighton University

Blocks High Blood Pressure: Calcium may save you from high blood pressure as you get older and is particularly effective in older people, notably those who are salt sensitive—blood pressure rises in response to eating too much sodium. In a recent review of all studies in which subjects with high blood pressure took calcium supplements, David A. McCarron, M.D., Oregon Health Sciences University, noted that the calcium tablets depressed blood pressure in 75 percent of the cases. It dropped an average 5 to 7 mm/Hg for systolic (upper number) and 3 to 4 mm/Hg for diastolic. The doses ranged from 400 milligrams to 2,000 milligrams daily and were usually taken for six to twelve weeks.

A high calcium intake may prevent the onset of high blood pressure in the first place. Investigators at Boston University Medical School recently tracked a large group of men for eighteen years. Those who ate the most calcium (up to 1,100 milligrams a day) were 20 percent less apt to develop high blood pressure as they aged than those eating the least (under 110 milligrams a day). Another study of nonoverweight, moderate drinkers under age forty showed that taking in 1,000 milligrams of calcium daily cut their risk of developing high blood pressure in later years by 40 percent.

If everyone took calcium supplements, blood pressure would drop in about 50 percent of Americans, says hypertension researcher Lawrence M. Resnick, M.D., of Wayne State University in Detroit. However, it would not change in 30 percent and it would rise in 20 percent, he says.

More remarkable, calcium may reverse some of high blood pressure's damage. Years of elevated blood pressure can result in strokes, left ventricular hypertrophy (enlargement of the left chamber of the heart) and congestive heart failure. Wayne State investigators found that taking a daily 1,000 milligrams of calcium carbonate for eight weeks caused enlarged hearts to diminish in size!

Inhibits Cancer: Another big plus for calcium: It can help thwart proliferation of cancer-prone cells. In a recent study, John Potter of the University of Minnesota found that 2,000 milligrams of calcium per day could normalize cell proliferation in the colons of men and women at high risk of colon cancer. This bears out numerous studies suggesting calcium has anticancer activity. For example, in animals calcium carbonate inhibits tumors by 23 to 44 percent; calcium chloride, by 30 to 35 percent; and calcium gluconate, by 19 to 41 percent. A study of humans

---

IT TAKES A LOT OF CALCIUM TO STAY YOUNG

Here's how much you need every day:
- ▲ Infants, birth to six months—400 milligrams.
- ▲ Infants, six months to one year—600 milligrams.
- ▲ Children, one to ten years—800 milligrams.
- ▲ Children and young adults, ages eleven through twenty-four—1,200 to 1,500 milligrams.
- ▲ Women, age twenty-five to fifty—1,000 milligrams.
- ▲ Men, age twenty-five and older—1,000 milligrams.
- ▲ Postmenopausal women—1,000 to 1,500 milligrams.
- ▲ Women over age sixty-five—1,500 milligrams.

—National Institutes of Health Expert Panel, 1994

---

revealed a three times greater risk of colon cancer among those eating the least dietary calcium compared with those eating the most calcium. If you're worried about colon cancer, the best calcium dose seems to be from 1,500 to 2,000 milligrams daily.

Fights Cholesterol: Surprisingly, calcium may be a weapon against bad cholesterol. In a test by Margo A. Denke, of the University of Texas Southwestern Medical Center in Dallas, men with moderately high cholesterol ate a diet fairly high in beef and fat and low in calcium—410 milligrams daily. Then they switched to a high-calcium regimen of 2,200 milligrams per day. Their average total cholesterol dipped 6 percent. More important, their artery-clogging bad LDL cholesterol fell 11 percent.

Why the calcium worked is fascinating. It partly blocked absorption of saturated fat in the gastrointestinal tract. Such animal fats from meat, cheese and butter are notorious at boosting cholesterol. If they are not absorbed, they can't raise cholesterol. Indeed, twice as much fat washed out in the men's stools during the high-calcium diets. You can't depend on calcium to cancel out the danger of a high-fat diet, but it may go a long way toward blunting its cholesterol-raising impact.

What About Food? Best sources of calcium are yogurt, milk, kale, broccoli, tofu, canned sardines and canned salmon with bones, and calcium-fortified foods, such as juice and bread. It takes several servings a day to get an antiaging dose.

An easy way to get calcium is to consume low-fat or nonfat milk and yogurt. A glass of skim milk contains 300 milligrams, a cup of nonfat yogurt, up to 415 milligrams, depending on the brand. Still, some nondairy foods are also good sources. In Asian countries, vegetables and tofu often provide enough calcium. Indeed, studies show you absorb more calcium from kale than from milk. However, you have to eat lots of kale to get as much calcium as you get in milk.

Twenty to 40 percent of Americans with mild to moderate hypertension would be able to either discontinue their antihypertensive medication or lower their dosages, just by getting adequate calcium. —Dr. David A. McCarron, Oregon Health Sciences University, Portland, Oregon

---

Do You Need a Supplement? Yes—unless you religiously eat several servings a day of high calcium foods, such as dairy products, canned sardines or salmon, leafy green vegetables, tofu or calcium-fortified foods. But, then again, why take chances? Calcium supplements are cheap, effective and reliable, says Harvard's Walter Willett. A separate tablet is needed because multivitamin-mineral pills do not contain nearly enough calcium. Even if you are on hypertension medication, calcium supplements can induce further drops in blood pressure, says Dr. McCarron. But he cautions, be sure to inform your physician if you start taking calcium supplements on top of medication.

How Much? For bone-protecting doses at various ages, see the chart (page 103). To prevent or correct other aging problems—high blood pressure, high cholesterol, cancer—you may need bigger doses of 1,000 to 2,000 milligrams of calcium per day.

What Kind? Don't take calcium supplements made of bone-meal or dolomite. They can contain dangerous amounts of

YOU CAN'T STAY YOUNG WITHOUT VITAMIN D

You need vitamin D to absorb calcium. Yet older Americans suffer "a silent epidemic of vitamin D deficiency," says Michael F. Holick, M.D., an endocrinologist at Boston University Medical Center. He says up to 40 percent of elderly people who break their hips lack vitamin D— mainly because aging skin is less able to make vitamin D from sunlight and aging kidneys are less able to convert the vitamin to the active type. Thus, without enough active vitamin D, bones grow weaker. A lack of vitamin D also makes women more vulnerable to breast cancer and men to prostate and colon cancer. Good food sources are vitamin D–fortified milk, liver, eel and fatty fish, such as salmon and sardines.

Older people who are rarely in the sun need 600 IU of vitamin D a day. If you get a lot of sun— you live in a sunny warm climate or you are exposed to sunlight a lot—200 IU of vitamin D daily, the amount in most multivitamin-mineral pills, is enough.

Using sunblock on your skin also blocks absorption of vitamin D, so if that's your practice, you may need a vitamin D supplement.

Caution: Don't consume excessive vitamin D. It's quite toxic. A toxic daily dose for adults could be as little as 2,000 IU, say experts.

lead. Best choices: calcium carbonate and calcium citrate. Be sure to check the label for the amount of pure or "elemental" calcium each tablet delivers. This tells the amount of usable calcium in the pill, and is the only way to know how much calcium you are really getting from a specific pill. Supplements differ greatly. For example, calcium gluconate contains only 9 percent elemental calcium; calcium carbonate has 40 percent. Tums are pure calcium carbonate, thus identical to a calcium supplement.

When to Take? You generally absorb 10 to 30 percent more from calcium supplements, notably from calcium carbonate, if you take them with a meal. But give yourself a time-out occasionally. Dr. Heaney advises cutting out the supplements for a week every three months or so to give your body time for bone remodeling, the process of releasing old bone and replacing it with new. If you keep taking 1,000 to 1,500 or more milligrams of calcium daily for long periods, there is never a dip that gives your body the cue to remodel.

How Much Is Too Much? Too much calcium might cause constipation. Drink lots of water, and space pills throughout day. Don't take more than 500 to 600 milligrams at one time for best absorption. If you're a postmenopausal woman taking estrogen replacement, you may need only 1,000 milligrams of calcium a day to keep bones safe.

Kids Alert! Youngsters are increasingly eating calcium-deficient diets because they substitute carbonated beverages for milk and because their parents often cut down on milk intake to avoid high fat. A better idea: Feed your kids low-fat or skim milk and other low-fat or nonfat dairy foods.

It's best that kids get calcium from foods, says Dr. Heaney, but if they don't, calcium supplements are called for.

> You need not get calcium exclusively from food or pills. Smartest antiaging practice: eat a high-calcium diet and take the entire recommended doses of calcium in supplements. It's never too late to buck up calcium, but for the best antiaging results, start before age twenty-five.

It's best to get your calcium from food. But it's better to get calcium in pills than not to get it at all. —Dr. David A. McCarron, Oregon Health Sciences University, and Dr. Robert Heaney, Creighton University

---

The Forgotten Antiaging Powerhouse

▲ ▲ ▲

(Why You Need Magnesium to Stop Aging)

Chances are great that you don't get enough magnesium to protect cells against premature aging. Thus, your heart is apt to give out at an earlier age, you are more apt to have a heart attack, your insulin levels are apt to go awry, your bones are more apt to break, and you're more apt to be plagued by chronic high blood pressure.

Don't risk aging prematurely and cutting your life short just because you don't get enough magnesium. It's a youth-preserving mineral, especially for your heart. Even small shortages of magnesium appear to make a difference in how long you live and how fast you age. For one thing, as you age you tend to eat diets lower in magnesium and worse, absorb less of it. That lack can accelerate the aging process, as animal studies strikingly illustrate. Animals made deficient in magnesium age more rapidly and die earlier. Depriving young animals of magnesium creates vascular changes and neuromuscular abnormalities typical in aged animals. Giving animals magnesium supplements prevents these premature aging changes. Indeed, animals starved of magnesium are nearly perfect specimens of accelerated aging, say French researchers.

If you chronically have suboptimal levels of magnesium, you, too, can expect to show the signs of old age earlier—in particular, clogged arteries, heart arrhythmias, (irregular heart beats), heart attacks, high blood pressure and insulin resistance possibily leading to diabetes.

THE ALARMING FACTS

▲ Only one in four Americans gets the recommended daily allowance for magnesium, even though the RDA is far too low to begin with, say many experts.
▲ Two-thirds of older people, who need it most, eat less than 75 percent of the RDA for magnesium.
▲ You're not likely to get enough magnesium from food unless you eat at least 2,000 calories a day.

HOW MAGNESIUM CAN FIGHT AGING

Curbs Free Radicals: Recent investigations by a team of scientists at the Center for Research on Human Nutrition at France's National Institute of Agricultural Research, suggest that the root cause of rapid aging induced by a magnesium deficiency is increased free radical activity in cells. They find cells from magnesium deficient animals more prone to free radical damage. Such cells' membranes become rigid, destroying cell integrity and disrupting the proper flow of calcium through membranes. This "uncontrolled calcium inflow," suspect French researchers, is a "central event in the aging process and cell injury."

Animals low in magnesium also release greater amounts of highly inflammatory agents called cytokines that in turn create more free radicals and subsequent cell damage. Long-term magnesium deficiency also robs the body of vitamin E, probably because so much is used up trying to fend off increased free radical attacks.

Worst of all the mitochondria, the energy factories of the cells particularly critical in heart function, are increasingly damaged in the absence of adequate magnesium. When you mess with mitochondria, you disrupt the very crux of a cell's life, the ability to create energy. Indeed, damage to cell mitochondria is considered the number one underlying cause of aging by free radical experts. The French investigators agree that free radical induced dysfunction in mitochondria is the primary cause of declining functions, thus premature aging, in magnesium deficient animals.

Saves Hearts: People who take in low amounts of magnesium are more apt to have heart disease, according to "about twenty worldwide population studies," says Ronald J. Elin, M.D., a magnesium authority at the National Institutes of Health. Magnesium seems to protect the heart several different ways, in particular by preventing spasms of the coronary arteries and abnormal heart rhythms that are a primary cause of sudden death. In one study of a cardiac unit, 53 percent of the patients had low magnesium. Indeed, the amount of magnesium in your body can help determine whether you live or die if you have a heart attack.

Further, magnesium helps deter formation of blood clots that help clog arteries and trigger heart attacks. Specifically, studies by Jerry L. Nadler, M.D., at City of Hope Medical Center in Duarte, California, show that magnesium inhibits release of thromboxane, a substance that makes blood platelets more sticky and apt to form clots. The mineral also tends to keep blood vessels from constricting, thus warding off rises in blood pressure, strokes and heart attacks. Magnesium has been so effective in regulating heartbeat and blood pressure that it

has been called "nature's calcium channel blocker," refer-
ring to prescription calcium blocker drugs used for those
purposes.

Lowers Blood Pressure: A major Harvard study found that
those getting low amounts of magnesium were more apt
to develop high blood pressure. A recent Swedish study
found a dramatic drop in blood pressure from taking
magnesium supplements. After nine weeks, systolic blood
pressure went down from 154 to 146 and diastolic pressure from 100 to 92 in patients taking about 360 milligrams of magnesium daily. In another study by Dutch
researchers at Erasmus University Medical School in Rot-
terdam, middle-aged and elderly women with mild to
moderate high blood pressure took magnesium supplements (485 milligrams a day) for six months. Their systolic blood pressure (upper number) fell 2.7 mm/Hg and
diastolic blood pressure fell 3.4 mm/Hg lower than that of
women taking a dummy pill.

Prevents and Reverses Diabetes: New evidence is popping
up linking diabetes with a deficiency of magnesium. Further, fairly low doses of magnesium may help prevent diabetic complications and intervene in the course of the
disease itself. The theory is that diabetics have a peculiar
defect in the metabolism of magnesium. Studies find that
most diabetics often have low levels of magnesium in
their cells and blood. This is worrisome, because a lack of
magnesium can enourage blood clotting, constriction of
blood vessels, high blood pressure, irregular heart beats
and insulin resistance, according to Robert K. Rude, M.D.,
associate professor of medicine at the University of
Southern California. He favors 300 to 400 milligram supplements daily, preferably of magnesium chloride, to cor-

rect diabetic deficiencies. Diabetes, he says, is characterized by magnesium depletion.

Postscript: Even if you don't have diabetes or heart disease, skimping on magnesium can make you more vulnerable to insulin resistance—a condition you don't want. In one study of normal healthy individuals, all developed a 25 percent greater insulin resistance on a magnesium-deficient diet. Such a sluggish abnormal functioning of insulin can eventually damage arteries and possibly bring on diabetes. (For more details on the hazards of insulin resistance, see page 281.)

Keeps Bones Strong: To maintain bone strength as you age you need magnesium, as well as calcium. The two work together, with vitamin D, to keep bones from deteriorating. Women prone to osteoporosis commonly lack magnesium. And a long-term deficiency of magnesium can help trigger osteoporosis, according to Mildred S. Seelig, M.D., adjunct professor of nutrition at the University of North Carolina. If you have low levels of magnesium, you are also apt to have low levels of active vitamin D needed to metabolize bone. This makes your bones doubly vulnerable to fractures.

Also, the ratio of calcium and magnesium is important. Too much calcium and too little magnesium makes your blood more apt to clot, possibly leading to strokes and heart attacks. You should get at least half as much magnesium as calcium, but many older Americans get only one-fourth as much magnesium as calcium, especially if they take calcium supplements. So, if you get 1,200 milligrams of calcium, as generally recommended, you need about 600 milligrams of magnesium. Additionally, the more fat and sugar you eat, the more magnesium you need, says Dr. Seelig.

THE ANTIAGING PROMISE OF MAGNESIUM

▲ Reduces vascular spasms
▲ Reduces angina (chest pain)
▲ Increases clot-busting activity
▲ Inhibits blood platelet stickiness leading to clots
▲ Helps keep heartbeats normal
▲ Boosts good types of blood cholesterol (HDLs and APO A1)
▲ Suppresses triglycerides
▲ Maintains normal bone structure
▲ Keeps free radicals away

Stretches Life: You're more apt to survive a heart attack if you don't skimp on magnesium. A recent ten-year study of 2,182 men in Wales found that those eating magnesium-low diets had one-and-a-half times the risk of sudden death from heart attacks as those eating one-third more magnesium. Also, the high-magnesium eaters were only half as likely to have any type of cardiovascular incident such as nonfatal heart attacks, strokes, angina (chest pain) or heart surgery. The protective average difference in magnesium intake was only an extra 30 milligrams—the amount in half an ounce of almonds.

What About Food? Actually, you can get lots of magnesium if you eat whole grains, nuts, seeds and legumes. You could get the current 300-milligram RDA dose from just a serving of bran cereal and nuts per day. Here's the magnesium per ounce in such foods: pumpkin and squash kernels, 152 milligrams; 100 percent bran cereal, 135 milligrams; almonds, 85 milligrams; filberts, 85 milligrams; cashews, 74 milligrams; pine nuts, 66 milligrams; peanuts, 51 milligrams; walnuts, 48 milligrams; oats, 42 milligrams; pecans, 37 milligrams; Cheerios, 39 milligrams; Wheaties, 31 milligrams; tofu, 29 milligrams; soybeans, 25 milligrams; lima beans, 15 milligrams.

Do You Need a Supplement? Decidedly yes, if you don't eat magnesium-rich foods. A supplement is necessary to retard premature aging.

How Much? A separate supplement of 200 to 300 milligrams seems to be an adequate antiaging dose, according to experts. Dr. Seelig insists that the total daily intake of magnesium should be about 500 milligrams. A typical multivitamin-mineral pill contains about 100 milligrams of magnesium or about 25 percent of the current RDA. So if you opt for more, you need a separate magnesium tablet.

What Type? Magnesium chloride, magnesium aspartate, magnesium gluconate and magnesium lactate all seem to be absorbed well and are better tolerated by most people than magnesium oxide.

How Much Is Too Much? More than 600 to 700 milligrams daily of elemental magnesium can cause diarrhea. A daily dose of 500 milligrams of elemental magnesium per day is considered extremely safe for the average individual with normal kidney function.

> *Warning: Don't take magnesium supplements if you have kidney problems or severe heart failure. And stop taking supplements if you develop diarrhea. If you have already had a heart attack, consult your physician before taking magnesium supplements.*

MAGNESIUM: NUTS' SECRET WEAPON?

One of the surprises revealed in recent research is that people who eat nuts have less heart disease. A study at Loma Linda (California) University found nuts to be the number one food among those most immune to heart disease. Enthusiastic nut eaters (at least five times a week) had about half the risk of heart attack and cardiovascular death as those who ate nuts less than once a week. Even snacking on a few nuts once a week seemed to reduce heart disease chances by one-fourth. There could be several reasons, including the good-type monounsaturated and omega-3 type oils in most nuts.

However, Ronald J. Elin, M.D., clinical pathologist at the National Institutes of Health, and an expert on magnesium, suggests that nuts' most powerful antiheart disease agent may be magnesium. Indeed, nuts are one of the richest sources of magnesium—namely, almonds, hazelnuts (filberts), cashews, pine nuts, peanuts, walnuts, pecans.

The Unique Mineral
That Keeps You Young

▲ ▲ ▲

(Why You Need Selenium to Stop Aging)

If you don't get enough selenium, your cells fall prey to viruses, cancer, heart disease and other signs of rapid aging. To keep your youth, take a low-level selenium supplement, as many research scientists do.

Imagine an agent that can keep vicious viruses, including the AIDS virus, from breaking out of cells and spreading death and destruction. That's selenium—a powerhouse antioxidant and essential trace mineral with diverse anti-aging properties. When your cells get low in selenium—as they tend to do with age—your immune functioning goes awry and you are more apt to fall prey to infections, cancer and heart disease. Further, selenium is not only an antioxidant on its own, it is an essential building block for the creation of glutathione peroxidase, one of the body's most critical enzymes that neutralizes free radicals, particularly those that attack fat molecules, literally turning them rancid. Some researchers believe much of selenium's antiaging power is due to its ability to boost production of this free radical–fighting glutathione enzyme.

The Alarming Facts

▲ As you age, your levels of selenium fall. Selenium blood levels dropped 7 percent after age sixty and 24 percent after age seventy-five, according to Italian research.

▲ Declining selenium signifies less antioxidant activity in your blood and tissues.

▲ People with low levels of selenium have more heart disease, cancer and arthritis.

How Selenium Can Fight Aging

Blocks Cancer: "Selenium is a powerful chemopreventive agent," says Dr. Donald J. Lisk, a selenium expert at Cornell University. In animals, selenium blocks up to 100 percent of various types of tumors. Throughout the world, people who have low blood levels of selenium and eat diets low in selenium tend to have more cancers of the breast, colon, liver, skin, lung and trachea. A recent study of seventeen hundred elderly Americans by University of Arizona investigators found that those with low blood levels of selenium were much more apt to have polyps, small growths that can lead to colon cancer. In fact, one-third of those with polyps had the lowest blood selenium. Only 9 percent with the highest blood selenium had polyps. So promising is the anticancer potential of selenium that it is now being tested in doses of 200 micrograms per day in human clinical trials to see if it prevents colon and skin cancer.

Indeed, selenium was one of the antioxidant supplements that slashed the cancer death rate in National Cancer Institute studies in Linxian, China. Selenium may be particularly important in preventing lung cancer. A recent large-scale Dutch study involving about three thousand older persons found that getting high levels of selenium in the diet cut the chances of lung cancer in half.

Selenium appears to fight cancer by preventing mutations, repairing damage to cells and boosting immune functions.

Reduces Heart Disease: Low blood levels of selenium make you more vulnerable to heart disease, studies show. A large-scale Finnish study found that those with the lowest blood levels of selenium were three times more apt to die of heart disease than those with the highest blood levels of selenium. Another study found that the lower your blood selenium, the greater the degree of blockage in arteries as determined by angiograms (heart X rays). Apparently, selenium can save your heart in several ways. It protects arteries by preventing platelet aggregation that tends to form blood clots, triggering heart attacks and strokes. Selenium also helps block oxidation of bad-type LDL cholesterol, thought to be the primary step in artery clogging.

Adequate selenium intake is unquestionably necessary if one is to attain optimal health and full life span potential. —Sheldon Saul Hendler, M.D., Ph.D., University of California, San Diego

---

Rejuvenates Immunity: Taking selenium can help bring your failing immunity back up to younger and healthier levels. So discovered researchers at the University of Brussels. They gave elderly subjects either 100 micrograms of selenium or a dummy pill for six months. Not surprisingly, selenium caused blood levels of the mineral to jump—nearly doubling within two months. Most important, lymphocyte response to mitogens—a marker of immune functions—which was low in the elderly, soared

ANTIAGING SECRETS OF THE EXPERTS

Donald J. Lisk: Noted Authority on Selenium
Professor of Toxicology at Cornell University

Dr. Lisk takes a supplement of 100 micrograms of selenium and eats two to four selenium-packed Brazil nuts every day.

79 percent, up to levels typically found in younger and healthier people.

Fights Viruses: Selenium can help keep viruses under control, according to remarkable new studies by U.S. Department of Agriculture researchers. They found that a normally harmless virus turned virulent, causing severe heart muscle damage, in mice raised on diets deficient in selenium or vitamin E. Without enough vitamin E and selenium, antioxidant defenses were weak, enabling the virus to undergo a mutation that turned it from Dr. Jekyll into Mr. Hyde, said researchers Orville A. Levander of the USDA and Melinda A. Beck of the University of North Carolina. The virus did not break out and damage the hearts of mice eating diets adequate in selenium and vitamin E. Researchers suspect a lack of selenium might similarly unleash the rage of many other viruses.

Curbs AIDS: Selenium, indeed, may be a key to the spread of AIDS. Low levels of selenium have been found in many AIDS patients. Now it's suspected the AIDS virus slowly depletes the body of selenium, and when the selenium is exhausted, the virus breaks out of an infected cell in search of more supplies, thus spreading the infection by attacking healthy cells, according to Will Taylor of the University of Georgia College of Pharmacy. Supplements of selenium might help contain the virus, he says, and prolong survival in AIDS patients.

What happens theoretically is this: In the presence of selenium, the virus actually makes a protein to repress its own replication. But when selenium gets low, the virus says it's time to switch on replication genes and get out of this cell to find more selenium elsewhere. "As long as there is enough selenium around in the cells, the virus behaves itself. When the selenium is depleted, then the virus can switch into a high rate of replication and cause full-blown AIDS," said Gerhard Schrauzer, emeritus professor of biochemistry at the University of California, San Diego. That selenium can help curb such a virulent virus is almost mind-boggling, say experts, and has consequences for all types of viral diseases.

Relieves Anxiety: If you're anxious about aging, selenium may relieve that, too. Taking 100 micrograms of selenium a day made subjects less anxious, depressed and tired after five weeks, according to a double-blind study of fifty healthy men and women by psychologists David Benton and Richard Cook at University College in Swansea, Wales. The mood of selenium takers improved dramatically, and those most deficient in selenium improved the most, notably in levels of anxiety. In other studies, elderly people given selenium plus vitamin E or other antioxidants experienced significant improvements in mood and mental functioning as well as increased blood flow to the brain.

THE ANTIAGING NUT

Eating a Brazil nut is just like taking a selenium pill. That is, if you buy Brazil nuts that are still in the shell, according to analyses at Cornell University. The average Brazil nut in the shell contains about 100 micrograms of selenium (the typical selenium tablet contains 50 or 100 micrograms). The reason: Imported nuts in the shells are grown in parts of the Brazilian jungle where the soil is highest in selenium. Imported Brazil nuts already shelled come from another part of Brazil where soil is lower in selenium; they average about 12 to 25 micrograms per nut, still a considerable dose.

What About Food? You get selenium in grains, sunflower seeds, meat, seafood—especially tuna, swordfish and oysters—and garlic. But for a major injection of selenium, nothing beats Brazil nuts, grown in the selenium-rich soil of the forests of the Amazon.

Do You Need a Supplement? Yes. And for anticancer protection, you need from 100 to 200 micrograms a day, says Dr. Lisk. He has also sampled the potency of many selenium supplements on the market and found them to be excellent. You don't have to worry that they deliver more than or less than the label claims, he says. Further, you probably need a separate pill, because you usually cannot get sufficient selenium in a typical multivitamin-mineral supplement.

How Much Is Too Much? Selenium can be toxic (hair loss, liver damage, joint inflammation) in high doses, so don't overdose on supplements. Even excessively eating

Brazil nuts could be toxic to the liver, as animal experiments have shown. But to get a toxic effect, you would have to eat as much as 2,500 micrograms of selenium a day, says Dr. Lisk. Japanese fishermen get over 500 micrograms a day without apparent harm. Inhabitants in China have developed severe toxic symptoms after 5,000 micrograms of selenium a day. Still, there is no reason to go above an antiaging dose of 200 micrograms per day, which experts say is safe.

The Master Antioxidant

▲ ▲ ▲

(Why You Need Glutathione to Stop Aging)

You must get your levels of glutathione up if you want to keep your youth and live longer. High blood levels of glutathione predict good health as you age and a long life. Low levels predict early disease and death.

God forbid that your cells should lose their zest for making an antioxidant substance called glutathione. But, alas, they do slack off as you age, weakening your resistance to free radical damage and exposing you to disease and premature aging. Glutathione is one of the most fascinating antioxidants, a naturally occurring amino acid that is in your diet and is also produced by your cells internally as part of the body's magnificently designed detoxification system to fend off free radical damage.

Indeed, glutathione is the most powerful, versatile and important of these self-generated antioxidants. "It is the master antioxidant," proclaims John T. Pinto of Memorial Sloan Kettering Cancer Center in New York. Glutathione is the body's main powerhouse for defusing and disposing of free radicals that bring on the woes of aging. It protects every cell, tissue and organ in the body. Further, it may determine the rate at which you age and your susceptibility to chronic diseases.

CAUTION: RAPID AGING AHEAD

A lack of glutathione in cells is a primary *cause* of faster aging, theorizes Calvin Lang, a professor of biochemistry at the University of Louisville. His message after forty years of research on glutathione is blunt: If you have lots of glutathione in your blood and tissues, you live longer and better; if you don't, your functioning declines dramatically as you age and you die earlier. In one experiment, Dr. Lang extended the life span of mosquitoes about 40 percent by feeding them chemicals that boosted glutathione tissue levels 50 to 100 percent.

Dr. Lang and Dr. Mara Julius, at the University of Michigan, more recently identified glutathione as a strikingly accurate biomarker in the blood, distinguishing healthy people over age sixty from those with disease. Subjects with 20 percent higher blood glutathione had only one-third the rates of arthritis, high blood pressure, heart disease, circulatory symptoms, diabetes, stomach symptoms and urinary tract infections as those with lower glutathione. "Even in very old age, people with the highest levels of glutathione bounce back from diseases and accidents the same way much younger people do," says Dr. Julius. "They are just more vigorous."

Glutathione's main antiaging powers? It regenerates immune cells. Explains Dr. Julius, "If you deplete glutathione, the cell disintegrates and loses its immune activity. If you add glutathione to that ailing cell, it regenerates and becomes immuno-efficient."

THE ALARMING FACTS

▲ Your blood levels of glutathione drop about 17 percent between ages forty and sixty.

GLUTATHIONE AT A GLANCE

Glutathione is made up of three amino acids and is produced in all cells of the body. Its main purpose is to break down and dispose of potentially dangerous toxins that invade your body. It is an antioxidant that cleanses fatty foods of free radical hazards in the digestive tract and protects cells everywhere against free radical harm. Because glutathione is a natural substance, it is also found in certain foods. Additionally, glutathione has been synthesized and made into supplements. Therefore, you can combat aging both by eating glutathione in food and by taking it as a supplement. Further, you can rev up your blood levels of glutathione by ingesting certain vitamins and other compounds that are building blocks the body uses to synthesize glutathione.

▲ If you have low glutathione, you are one-third more likely to have chronic diseases, a sense of poor health, decreased functions and early death.

▲ Fully 77 percent of people hospitalized with chronic diseases had a glutathione deficiency, in one study.

▲ Eating fat boosts your need for glutathione; thus the more fat you eat, the greater your expected deficiency of glutathione.

How Glutathione Can Fight Aging

Rejuvenates Immunity: A drop in cell levels of glutathione as we age allows free radical activity to heat up unchecked, causing a gradual decay of immune functioning. Yet, by replenishing glutathione, you can abort and reverse this "inevitability." When Tufts researcher Dr. Simin Meydani added glutathione to the white blood cells of elderly people, immune activity revved up, nearly equaling that of cells of much younger people. Specifically, glutathione boosts the ability of cells to divide, enabling them to mount stronger attacks on foreign invaders.

How utterly devastating shortages of glutathione can be to cells was dramatically illustrated by experiments at Stanford University School of Medicine. When deprived of 25 percent of their normal glutathione, T-cells (the warriors of the immune system) of healthy individuals became so disturbed, they could no longer appropriately respond to signals to wage war on microbes. The famished cells eventually became so confused that they actually killed themselves, a phenomenon researchers call "programmed cell death."

Postscript: Glutathione has such a powerful effect that in test tubes it stops the replication or spread of the AIDS virus by about 90 percent. AIDS patients are typically low in glutathione. Thus, the antioxidant is being tested on HIV patients to see if it can partially restore immune functioning.

Blocks General Cell Damage: Glutathione is the Rambo that rushes in to save your cells by neutralizing and breaking down free radicals so they are harmlessly flushed out of the body. It can deactivate at least thirty cancer-causing substances, according to Dean Jones, Ph.D., associate professor of biochemistry at Emory University School of Medicine. Glutathione even acts as a prophylactic against the formation of free radicals by destroying peroxides that are parents to free radicals. Glutathione's formidable powers as a free radical terminator may help explain why eating fruits and vegetables, naturally high in glutathione, is so often tied to lower rates of cancer, heart disease and other chronic diseases. In a recent study, people who ate the most glutathione-rich raw fruits and vegetables were only half as likely to develop oral cancer as those eating the least.

Busts Up Dangerous Fat: Especially spectacular, gluta-thione can help save you from the awful consequences of eating dangerous rancid fats. Glutathione actually detoxi-fies or "cleanses" food of oxidized or rancid fat in your intestinal tract, preventing it from detonating into showers of free radicals to attack your cells. In a striking study, Tak Yee Aw, Ph.D., associate professor of physiology at the Louisiana State University Medical Center, put oxidized fat into animals' intestinal tracts. When she added glutathione, the amounts of free radicals that were metabolized and released from intestinal cells into the bloodstream fell dra-matically. "The moment rancid fat enters the cells," explains Dr. Aw, "glutathione destroys it. If there is enough glutathione to destroy all the rancid fat that enters, none is left to go back out to circulate through the blood." But if your cells in the GI tract have too little glutathione and you eat too much rancid fat, or both, the defense collapses, releasing hazardous oxidized fat to circulate throughout your body, promoting all the torments of aging.

Prevents and Cures Diabetes: In an exciting breakthrough, researchers at Duke University Medical Center actually cured Type II (adult-onset) diabetes in animals by boosting glutathione levels. In the experiment, diabetes-prone mice on high-fat diets developed diabetes. The

THE ANTIAGING PROMISE OF GLUTATHIONE

Here's what glutathione promises to do to keep you young:

▲ Maintain healthy immune functioning.
▲ Rejuvenate old and weak immune systems.
▲ Help save you from cancer.
▲ Prevent injury to lungs due to free radicals.
▲ Flush free radicals out of rancid fat you eat.
▲ Keep blood cholesterol from becoming oxidized and toxic.
▲ Help cure some forms of Type II diabetes.
▲ Help prevent macular degeneration, an age-related eye disease.

reason, explains Duke biochemist Emmanuel Opara: When mice burned the gobs of dietary fat, high amounts of oxygen free radicals were generated. These radicals "interfered with or shut off the body's ability to metabolize sugar. This led to an overload of sugar in the blood, causing the diabetes."

Incredibly, the diabetes disappeared when mice were fed glutamine, a natural amino acid that caused levels of glutathione to skyrocket. The glutathione then mopped up the destructive free radicals so they no longer hindered sugar metabolism. Sugar blood levels fell. This gives Dr. Opara and colleagues hope that antioxidants may also delay or eliminate such diabetes in humans. Tests are under way to find out.

Your blood level of glutathione tells you the difference between chronological and functional age. Those who have high levels of glutathione are healthier and younger. —Dr. Mara Julius, University of Michigan epidemiologist

———————————

How Does It Work? Glutathione fights aging through at least two major pathways—your gut and your bloodstream. One: When you eat glutathione, as in food or supplements, it gets into the cells of your gastrointestinal tract and sets up a fat-detoxification system on the site, blocking an exportation of hazardous oxidized fat throughout your body. However, how much glutathione gets to other parts of the body intact is uncertain, because digestive juices break down glutathione into other substances. Thus, glutathione from foods and supplements may not reach the bloodstream and other tissues and organs in sufficient amounts to make a major difference.

Two: You can boost glutathione in your blood and consequently in all other tissues *indirectly* by consuming chemical building blocks that form glutathione in the body. For example, vitamin C and selenium boost blood levels of glutathione, as does glutamine—an amino acid supplement.

How to Get More Antiaging Glutathione in Your Cells

Eat Glutathione-Foods with Every Meal: They are antidotes to wholesale cellular destruction that can follow eating peroxided or rancid polyunsaturated fats. Most glutathione-rich are fresh and frozen fruits and vegetables; cooking and heat-processing destroys glutathione. An analysis by Emory's Dr. Jones showed that fresh and frozen raw fruits and vegetables have about eight times more glutathione than canned fruits and vegetables. Cooking and grinding up or juicing foods also destroys some glutathione. For example, raw carrots had 75 milligrams of glutathione per 100 grams of dry weight. But cooked fresh carrots had 35 milligrams and canned carrots had none! Similarly, raw tomato juice had 169 milligrams of glutathione; canned juice had 27 milligrams. Fresh raw spinach had 166 milligrams, cooked fresh spinach, 108 milligrams and canned spinach, 27 milligrams.

Except for orange juice, fruit juices had little glutathione. Walnuts are high in glutathione. Fresh meats also contain high glutathione but have other health drawbacks.

Eat Cruciferous Vegetables: Brussels sprouts, cabbage, cauliflower and broccoli (cruciferous vegetables) possess several compounds that keep your cells awash in antioxidant glutathione. University of Illinois scientists Matthew A. Wallig and Elizabeth H. Jeffery discovered a strong glutathione-booster, called cyanohydroxybutene (CHB) in cruciferous vegetables. When rats ate CHB (equivalent to eating a pound of Brussels sprouts for humans), glutathione levels in their pancreatic cells tripled in four days. Protective glutathione in liver cells doubled within three days.

Additionally, cruciferous vegetables contain sulforaphane and iberin, two other chemicals that spur internal production of glutathione. Plus, broccoli has high concentrations of preformed glutathione.

Take Vitamin C: Taking at least 500 milligrams per day of vitamin C is a quick, easy way to be sure cells maintain high levels of glutathione. As a test, researchers at Arizona

---

FRUITS AND VEGETABLES
HIGHEST IN GLUTATHIONE

COMMON SERVING	MILLIGRAMS
Avocado, raw	31.3
Watermelon, raw	28.3
Asparagus, fresh cooked	26.3
Grapefruit, raw, peeled	14.6
Acorn squash, baked	14.4
Potatoes, boiled with skin	12.7
Strawberries, frozen	11.9
Okra, fresh cooked	11.1
Tomatoes, raw	10.9
Orange raw, peeled	10.6
Cantaloupe, raw	9.4
Cauliflower, fresh cooked	8.2
Broccoli spears, fresh cooked	7.8
Peaches, raw, peeled	6.8
Onions, fresh cooked	6.7
Zucchini squash, fresh cooked	6.5
Carrots, raw	5.9
Spinach, raw	5.0

Source: Dean Jones, Emory University

State University at Tempe gave healthy men and women doses of 500 milligrams of vitamin C daily for two weeks and 2,000 milligrams for another two weeks. Glutathione in red blood cells jumped an average 50 percent after the 500-milligram dose and did not rise further on the higher dose. But you must keep taking the vitamin C; glutathione dropped within a week after vitamin C was discontinued. In another study, glutathione plunged 50 percent in men who ate less than 60 milligrams of vitamin C daily, the amount in one orange.

Take Glutamine: Oddly, taking an amino acid supplement, glutamine, is apt to boost your blood levels of glutathione much better than taking in glutathione directly. Glutamine prods your liver to synthesize quantities of glutathione, according to Harvard researchers. How much glutathione rises is uncertain and depends greatly on individual factors, including whether glutathione stores are low. When Harvard investigators fed glutamine to animals low in glutathione, blood levels of glutathione jumped about 40 percent. Interestingly, survival rates rose by the same percentage. In another study of humans with inflammation, blood glutathione rose about 20 percent after subjects took 5,000 to 15,000 milligrams of glutamine daily. (For other antiaging things glutamine does, see page 135.)

Take Selenium and Eat Brazil Nuts: Selenium supplements and foods high in selenium, such as Brazil nuts, also stimulate increased bodily production of glutathione. Indeed, increased glutathione activity, some scientists believe, is a primary reason selenium inhibits cancer in laboratory animals and may do the same in humans.

Take Glutathione: If you can't be sure that you get enough glutathione-rich fruits and vegetables, it makes sense to take 100 milligrams of glutathione with your main meal as insurance. The reason: Glutathione helps detoxify oxidized fat, blocking the intestinal tract's absorption of dam-

ANTIAGING SECRETS OF THE EXPERTS
Bruce Ames, Ph.D.:
Famed Biochemist and Antioxidant Expert

Dr. Ames, professor of molecular biology at the University of California at Berkeley, is world-renowned for his pioneering research on free radicals and antioxidants. He thinks they are the key to aging. To lengthen your life span, he advises eating fruits and vegetables and not smoking. He also takes daily doses of:

▲ Vitamin C—250 to 500 milligrams.
▲ Vitamin E—400 IU.
▲ Multi-vitamin-mineral tablet.

"In the next hundred years we're going to see life expectancy go way up. People will routinely be living to one hundred, and well beyond."

aging free radicals so they aren't transported around your body. You may also get some small boosts of glutathione in your blood from supplements, although one study showed that taking 3,000 milligrams of glutathione daily did not significantly raise glutathione blood levels. Note: You must take the glutathione pills with meals to blunt the effects of bad fat and to have a significant antioxidant, antiaging effect.

How Much? From 25 to 50 milligrams a day of glutathione, available in food, is enough to detoxify dangerous fatty elements in a meal, according to calculations by Emory's Dr. Dean Jones. He eats foods containing about 100 milligrams of glutathione a day.

How Much Is Too Much? Experts, such as Dr. Jones, see no danger in megadoses of thousands of milligrams of glutathione a day. Such megadoses have been used in human studies without detectable side effects, he says.

Can You Have Your Blood Tested for Glutathione? Unfortunately, blood tests for glutathione are not readily available. Reliable blood tests have been only recently developed and are currently used almost exclusively in research projects.

WHO NEEDS GLUTAMINE? YOU DO—MAYBE

Glutamine is an amino acid supplement that pumps up glutathione. That alone makes glutamine an awesome antiaging agent. But it does far more, say Douglas Wilmore, M.D., professor of surgery at Harvard Medical School, and his physician wife, Judy Shabert, author of *The Ultimate Nutrient Glutamine*. Dr. Wilmore has done research on glutamine and says it's an essential supplement for anyone who is ill or under stress. Glutamine strengthens immunity, cuts short illness and hastens recovery, he has found. Remarkably, glutamine also actually rejuvenates muscles weakened by stress and illness. Dr. Wilmore says if you are sick, or under stress, glutamine is the one nutrient that must be added to your diet—and yes, aging may be considered a form of stress. At

Harvard's Brigham and Women's Hospital, giving about 30,000 milligrams of glutamine to critically ill surgical patients is fairly routine.

Although totally healthy people may not need extra glutamine, its antioxidant qualities make it a suitable anti-aging supplement in some circumstances. Dr. Wilmore, age fifty-six, who is in excellent health and runs about forty miles a week, takes two teaspoons of glutamine powder daily (8,000 milligrams) and twice that much if he has an infection. (Duke University's Dr. Emmanuel Opara, who used glutamine to boost glutathione in diabetic mice, also routinely takes 2,000 milligrams of glutamine as a general health supplement.)

It seems the full muscles you had in youth are irretrievable, although this situation need not develop. If people would supply their bodies with glutamine in times of stress, they could prevent muscle from wasting away. Glutamine levels must be normal before muscle can be regenerated. —Dr. Judy Shabert, author of *The Ultimate Nutrient Glutamine*

Glutamine powder is preferable to tablets; the powder is tasteless and dissolves readily in liquid. You can mix it in water, applesauce or cold puddings, suggests Dr. Shabert. Don't combine it with highly acidic foods such as vinegar or with hot foods. It's okay to dissolve glutamine powder in citrus juice if you drink it immediately. Both heat and acid destroy glutamine, although stomach acid does not adversely affect absorption of glutamine. A typical 50- to 500-milligram tablet of glutamine probably is too low a dose to do much good and is relatively expensive compared to glutamine powder, says Dr. Shabert.

Glutamine appears absolutely safe, even in high doses. Daily doses of up to 40,000 milligrams, taken under the supervision of a physician, have produced no noticeable adverse effects, says Dr. Wilmore.

Caution: If you are ill, take glutamine only with a doctor's supervision.

Amazing New Aging Terminator

▲ ▲ ▲

(How Coenzyme Q-10 Can Stop Aging)

If you want extra insurance against growing old prematurely, take supplements of coQ-10, as many researchers do. It helps correct deficiencies that come with age, particularly related to your heart, brain, immune functioning and general resistance to chronic diseases. And it could make you younger and friskier in old age.

Maybe you have never heard of an antioxidant known as coenzyme Q-10, ubiquinol-10 or vitamin Q. It is not exactly a household word—yet. But it's destined to be. It is being hailed by scientists as one of the brightest new antioxidants around for postponing aging and preventing or treating age-related diseases, namely heart disease. It's a natural substance produced by your body. It's also found in certain foods, notably seafood, and it's been synthesized into a supplement that is available at health food stores. It's unsure how much you need, but it seems certain that taking in more than your body produces may help defeat the ravages of aging and even prolong life. Thus you may be aging far too rapidly because your cells don't get enough coenzyme Q-10.

For anyone over age fifty or so, taking coenzyme Q-10 supplements could reenergize aging tissues, allevi-

ating the effects of the aging process and age-associated diseases. —Professor Anthony W. Linnane, Centre for Molecular Biology and Medicine, Monash University, Clayton, Australia

———————

Unfortunately, your body's production of coQ-10, as it is called, begins to decline around age twenty, often leaving you seriously deficient by middle age. The cells of aged and diseased hearts show grave deficiencies of coQ-10, suggesting that the surge in degenerative heart disease after age fifty is tied to drops in coQ-10. Just when the body needs it most to fight off aging diseases, coQ-10 production falls. The most sensible way to correct the matter: Take coQ-10 supplements. Once again, the ravages of aging seem greatly due to a deficiency of antioxidants, in this case, coQ-10.

How CoQ-10 Works

Nobody is sure of the many ways coQ-10 fights aging. But here's what scientists do know. CoQ-10 is an antioxidant, similar to vitamin E, that protects fat molecules from becoming oxidized or infused with free radicals that go on rampages and irreparably damage cells. CoQ-10 helps stabilize cell membranes, vital in keeping all cells intact, functional and alive. But some say coQ-10's greatest talents are displayed in the tiny energy factories of the cells, called mitochondria, where oxygen is burned to give cells energy to carry on the business of life, a process called bioenergetics. CoQ-10 is often called the "spark" that starts the mitochondrial engines, without which cell life, and thus human life, ceases to exist.

It's easy to grasp why coQ-10 and other antioxidants are so essential to keeping your youth when you understand that aging accelerates in direct proportion to the amount of free radical damage to the mitochondrial power stations. Such damage shuts down cells' power supplies by as much as 80 percent, according to Dr. Bruce Ames. These power shortages drastically impair the functioning of the heart, liver and brain, studies show. In other words, the energy grows weak, the bio-electricity goes down, the lights go dim or out. Replenishing lost supplies of coQ-10 may help stop that from happening.

CoQ-10, not surprisingly, is highly concentrated in heart muscle cells, which need tremendous amounts of energy to keep a healthy heart pumping some one hundred thousand times per day. That may account for the fact that a lack of coQ-10 is particularly evident in a weakened heart.

I believe that cardiovascular disease may be very significantly caused by a deficiency of coQ-10. —Dr. Karl Folkers, University of Texas

---

How Coenzyme Q-10 Can Fight Aging

Saves Arteries: Coenzyme Q-10 strikes at the root cause of atherosclerosis. It is exceptionally strong in halting the relentless oxidation of blood cholesterol that is the first step in making a rotten mess of your arteries, precipitating heart attacks and strokes. According to Boston University researcher Balz Frei, ubiquinol-10 prevents artery-destroying oxidation of LDL bad-type cholesterol much more efficiently than either vitamin E, which is an acknowledged antioxidant heavyweight in this arena, or beta carotene. However, coQ-10 is quickly consumed during this process, so having lots on hand is critical in keeping arteries unclogged and young. Since fatty fish is the best dietary source of coQ-10, this may help explain why fish eaters have healthier arteries.

I think ubiquinol-10 [coenzyme Q-10] is going to turn out to be just as important as vitamin E and C.
—Dr. Bruce N. Ames, leading antioxidant researcher, University of California at Berkeley

---

Revives Failing Hearts: Heart failure, also called cardiomyopathy—a potentially deadly weakening of heart muscle—is the number-one heart hazard in older people. The heart becomes enlarged and too weak to pump enough blood, often leaving its victim a cardiac cripple and a candidate for a heart transplant. A prime reason for our growing epidemic of heart failure is a widespread unsuspected deficiency of coQ-10, insists Karl Folkers, Ph.D., director of the Institute for Biomedical Research at the University of Texas at Austin, who has pioneered coQ-10 research since 1957. He has found one-fourth less coQ-10 in the blood of heart disease patients than in healthy individuals. He also detected serious coQ-10 deficiencies in the heart tissue of 75 percent of heart disease patients. He further showed that three-fourths of elderly patients with cardiomyopathy improved significantly after taking coenzyme Q-10.

Lowers Blood Pressure: Taking an average 225 milligrams of coQ-10 daily reduced blood pressure in about 85 percent of 109 patients with high blood pressure, according to a recent study by Texas cardiologist Peter Langsjoen, M.D., in cooperation with researchers at the University of Texas at Austin. CoQ-10 caused no blood pressure changes in 15 percent of patients, and one patient got worse. Gen-

OTHER COUNTRIES BET THEIR LIVES ON IT

CoQ-10 has been used for decades in other countries to treat the chronic diseases of aging, mainly heart failure. It's been prescribed for more than forty million heart patients worldwide, and is approved in Japan and Europe for the treatment of congestive heart failure.

Israel: In Israeli hospitals, says Dr. Ya'acov Gindin, head of the Geriatric Educational and Research Institute at Kaplan Hospital in Jerusalem, "coenzyme Q-10 is routinely given by cardiology departments to patients with congestive heart failure."

Italy: It's been widely tested in Italy in multicenter trials involving 2,500 patients. Fully 80 percent of 1,113 heart failure patients, average age sixty-nine, improved by taking 100 milligrams of coQ-10 daily along with conventional therapy. A follow-up study showed that 50 milligrams of coQ-10 per day for four weeks—either alone or with other treatments—also significantly improved symptoms of heart failure and quality of life. Further, Italian investigators reported that coQ-10 in a double-blind trial dramatically reduced hospitalization and serious complications of chronic congestive heart failure.

Sweden: Swedish investigators recently found that low blood levels of coQ-10 predicted death in heart patients. Among a group of ninety-four randomly chosen hospital patients over age fifty, those who died within six months had lower levels of coQ-10 than survivors. A recent survey found that about 15 percent of Swedes and 20 percent of Danes take coQ-10 supplements.

Japan: Japanese researchers began testing coQ-10 for congestive heart failure in the 1960s, completing twenty-five studies, including two large double-blind trials by 1976. The results showed improvement in about 70 percent of the patients. By 1987, more than ten million Japanese were taking coQ-10 as a prescription drug for cardiac problems. Japan controls the making and marketing of coQ-10. It is synthesized and produced by several Japanese companies, then exported to supplement distributors and packagers in various countries, including the United States.

---

erally, however, taking coQ-10 pushed systolic (upper number) pressure down from 159 to 147, and diastolic pressure from 94 to 85, usually within three or four months. Further, echocardiograms (heart ultrasound pictures) found improvements in heart function. Most important, at the start of the study nearly all patients were on antihypertensive drugs. After coQ-10 treatment, 51 percent of the patients were able to completely stop taking from one to three of their antihypertensive medications and 25 percent were able to control their blood pressure with coQ-10 alone.

CoQ-10 is remarkable stuff. People feel so much better after taking it. It makes such a dramatic improvement, it's unthinkable for me to practice medicine without it. —Dr. Peter Langsjoen, cardiologist and coenzyme Q-10 researcher in Tyler, Texas

---

Boosts Immune Functioning: One way coenzyme Q-10 fights aging is by stimulating immunity or erasing an immunodeficiency. For example, older mice produce only one-third the antibodies against foreign invaders as young mice. But when elderly mice are given coQ-10, their anti-body production jumps two and a half fold, bringing them up to 80 percent the antibody production of young mice. It happens in humans, too. Immunoglobulin or antibody G (IgG), the major antibody in the blood, rose significantly in patients receiving oral doses of 60 milligrams of coQ-10 daily, in studies by Dr. Folkers. The jumps usually happened between one and three months after the treatment began.

Protects Brain from Damage: Some researchers speculate that coQ-10, because of its importance in protecting cells' mitochondria, might help prevent degenerative brain dis-ease, such as Alzheimer's disease, Lou Gehrig's disease, and gradual loss of memory and brain functioning, all too often considered "normal" in old age. The mitochondria are prime targets of free radical damage in brain cells, leading to decline in mental function, says leading free radical researcher Dr. Denham Harman, University of Nebraska. Coenzyme Q-10 is thought to be one of the few known antioxidants that can penetrate and restore vitality to the mitochondria.

Prolongs Youth and Life: Mice on a regimen of coenzyme Q-10 stay younger longer. Most spectacular, they remain extremely active in old age compared with mice not getting coQ-10, according to recent studies at UCLA by pathologist Steven B. Harris, M.D. Such mice also "look terrific, their coats are better, they groom themselves better—they look a few months younger," says L. Stephen Coles, M.D., Ph.D., of the California Institute of Technology, an expert on coQ-10 and other antiaging substances. But interestingly, the coQ-10 advantages did not show up until the mice became old; there was little difference in young mice on coQ-10. Notes Dr. Coles: "Halfway through life all the mice look alike. But when they get to the very end of their life span, the differences suddenly jump out at you. The coQ-10 mice begin to look better and better." Also, 30 percent of the coQ-10 mice lived about two months longer than noncoQ-10 mice, in the UCLA studies. But coQ-10 did not create new records for mice life spans.

Both Dr. Harris and Dr. Coles, as well as UCLA professor of gerontology Roy Walford, take about 30 milligrams a day of coQ-10 as a prophylactic against aging.

You should not start taking coQ-10 on grounds that you're going to instantly *look better, feel better and be happier. CoQ-10 is an insurance policy, an investment in the future, and the payoff will only happen at the end of life.* —Dr. L. Stephen Coles, California Institute of Technology

---

Do You Need a Supplement? It's good antiaging insurance, especially if you are fifty or over and likely to be low in coenzyme Q-10. If you have a decline in heart function, it's even more important.

How Much? Thirty milligrams a day is a common antiaging dose if you are generally healthy. People with signs of chronic disease need higher doses; typical is 50 to 150 milligrams. Dr. Langsjoen has found that 120 milligrams twice a day for a total of 240 milligrams raises blood coQ-10 to levels consistent with optimum heart functioning in 80 percent of heart failure patients. CoQ-10 stays in the blood a very long time. Studies show that coQ-10 reaches its maximum high level in blood after a single dose of 100 milligrams. Thus, it's okay to take 100 or 200 milligrams at one time, says Dr. Langsjoen, instead of dividing the doses.

Caution: Do not replace current medication with coQ-10 except on a doctor's advice. In cases of illness, including congestive heart failure, coQ-10 is generally used with drug therapy, not in place of it. You need medical follow-up to monitor improvement in heart function and possible adjustments in medication. If you are taking drugs for specific conditions, consult with your physician about adding coQ-10.

What Type? All coQ-10 sold in the United States is made in Japan. It comes in pressed tablets, powder-filled capsules and oil-based gelcaps. Oil-based capsules and chewable tablets are especially good because they are readily absorbed, says Dr. Langsjoen. Some companies make flavored chewable wafers.

Important: Always take coQ-10 tablets with a little fat—such as peanut butter or olive oil—or in an oil-based capsule. Otherwise it is not absorbed well, and tablets swallowed with water have been known to pass through the body totally intact, delivering no benefit.

How Soon Does It Take Effect? As a general antioxidant, coQ-10 kicks in almost immediately to protect cells, but you're not likely to notice any benefits—any more than you would from doses of other antioxidant vitamins, such as E or C. However, if you have a severe deficiency, you might have benefits as quickly as a few days. Generally, the improvement in heart patients is gradual, becoming evident in one to three months or longer, according to Dr. Folkers.

How Much Is Too Much? Are there side effects? "No," says Dr. Coles, "there is no downside to taking coQ-10." Coenzyme Q-10 is deemed one of the safest substances ever tested. Even at very high doses, no significant toxicity in animal or long-term human studies has been recorded, says Dr. Folkers. The only noticeable, but very rare, side effect from oral doses of coQ-10 has been mild transient nausea.

What About Food? Studies on foods containing coQ-10 are not comprehensive. But top sources are fatty fish, notably mackerel and sardines; organ meats such as heart, liver and kidney; beef; soy oil and peanuts. One pound of sardines or two and a half pounds of peanuts provide about 30 milligrams of coQ-10.

Some Other Ways to Boost CoQ-10

Take Vitamin E: Vitamin E may stimulate production of coQ-10, according to animal studies, suggesting another way both coQ-10 and vitamin E enhance immunity. In one study doses of vitamin E boosted coQ-10 in animal livers by 30 percent.

Get Enough Selenium: This trace mineral, even in tissues that are not deficient, also boosted biosynthesis of coQ-10, possibly helping account for selenium's reputation as a cancer fighter and heart protector.

Get Your B Vitamins: To make coQ-10, your body needs vitamin B6, B12, B2, niacin and folic acid.

The Brain-Saving Herb from Europe

▲   ▲   ▲

(Why You Need Ginkgo to Stop Aging)

If you have any kind of circulatory problem or want to avoid one, including fading mental faculties that can come with age, ginkgo is a good bet—just what the doctor might order if he or she knew about it. Luckily, you can find it on your own at any health food store.

Admittedly, ginkgo sounds strange to many Americans, like an exotic substance from the realm of the Teenage Mutant Ninja Turtles. But it's actually a very common ornamental tree growing throughout the United States as well as the rest of the world. Its leaf, pulverized into a powder or liquid, has long been revered for its antiaging effects on the brain. And after five thousand years of on-and-off medicinal popularity, ginkgo biloba, as the tree is called, is undergoing a monumental revival. Ginkgo is coming of age because it jibes with the needs of an aging population. Its antiaging powers have made a big scientific splash particularly in Germany and France, where tens of millions of people have used it with great success.

Ginkgo is "the most important" medicinal plant agent "to be marketed in Europe during the last decade," declares noted medicinal plant authority Varro E. Tyler,

Ph.D., at Purdue University. In Germany, for example, where the leaf extract has been rigorously tested, doctors write more than five million prescriptions a year for ginkgo, mainly to arrest and reverse some of the most dreaded symptoms of aging, including deteriorating memory.

WHAT IS GINKGO?

Technically, the antiaging agent is called extract of ginkgo biloba (EGb). Ginkgo is the name of a two-hundred-million-year-old large ornamental tree that still thrives in temperate climates throughout the world, including the United States. Its leaves—the medicinal part—are divided into two lobes, hence the name biloba. It takes about fifty pounds of dried leaves to make one pound of ginkgo biloba extract that is then used as a liquid or capsule, or is pressed into tablets.

GINKGO'S ANTIAGING SECRETS

Ginkgo's best-known antiaging trait, as reported in prestigious scientific journals, is its ability to improve blood circulation. This is critical to the elderly whose blood vessels are typically old, inflexible and clogged. Apparently, ginkgo encourages blood to squeeze through even the tiniest, narrowed vessels to nourish oxygen-starved tissue in the brain, heart and limbs, often restoring memory and wiping away muscle pain, among other things. More than three hundred scientific papers have been published on ginkgo, many confirming that ginkgo stimulates blood flow feeding oxygen to tissues, most likely by dilating blood vessels and discouraging blood platelets from sticking together and forming clots. Furthermore, ginkgo delivers healing oxygen and blood not only to the healthy areas of the brain, but specifically to disease-damaged areas, actually bringing new life to an aging brain.

Another source of ginkgo's power: It is a potent antioxidant. A recent test showed ginkgo even stronger than vitamin E in scavenging free radicals, thus blocking highly destructive oxidation of fatty cell membranes. Dr. K. Drieu of the Pasteur Institute in France attributes ginkgo's effect mainly to "a restoration of membrane integrity" following free radical attacks. In remarkable new animal studies, Dr. Drieu also finds that ginkgo can actually rejuvenate brain cells' ability to receive signals from neurotransmitters that direct brain functions. For example, ginkgo dramatically restored specific receptor sites on brain cells, increasing transmission of an all-important brain chemical, serotonin, that had been lost during aging. This is another thrilling way ginkgo may reverse aging's toll on the brain.

Ginkgo has earned a reputation for improving the quality of life for the elderly in Europe, and should be a part of the plan for anyone who hopes to live to a ripe and healthy old age. —Rob McCaleb, president, Herb Research Institute in Colorado, a nonprofit organization for the study of herbs

---

How Ginkgo Can Fight Aging

Improves Brain Functions: With age, the body's ability to get enough oxygenated blood through rigid narrowed capillaries of the brain often falters, contributing to a condition called cerebral insufficiency—a medical nicety for the dawning of senility. The signs are well-known: diminished concentration and short-term memory, increased absentmindedness, confusion, lack of energy, tiredness, depression, anxiety, dizziness, and tinnitus (ringing in the ears).

Unquestionably, ginkgo can ameliorate the symptoms of cerebral insufficiency, according to sterling research, including an analysis of forty controlled studies by Drs. Jos Kleijnen and Paul Knipschild at the University of Limburg in Maastricht, the Netherlands. Writing in the *British Journal of Clinical Pharmacology* in 1992, they concluded that the evidence for using ginkgo to treat cerebral insufficiency equals that for the pharmaceutical drug codergocrine (Hydergine™) commonly prescribed for cerebral insufficiency.

The Dutch doctors particularly cited two German studies done in 1991. One study of ninety-nine older patients who had suffered brain disturbances for slightly more than two years found that after three months, 72 percent taking ginkgo had improved compared with 8 percent given a placebo (dummy pill). Similarly, German researchers studied two hundred patients, average age sixty-nine, who had suffered memory problems for about four years. When they were given ginkgo for three months, memory improved in 71 percent, compared with 32 percent on placebo.

The Dutch researchers were so convinced of the value of ginkgo that they said they personally would take it if they had signs of cerebral insufficiency, especially since none of the studies found any clear or serious side effects. The typical effective daily dose for treating cerebral insufficiency in the studies: 120 milligrams daily.

Improvements are generally noticeable after four to six weeks.

The management of cerebral edema is one of the unsolved problems in neurology and neurosurgery, but ginkgo extract has proven effective in animal experiments to reduce chemically induced brain edema. It also protects the liver, reduces arrhythmias, inhibits potentially life-threatening constriction of the bronchi during allergic reactions, and is being evaluated for use in asthma, graft rejection, shock, stroke, organ preservation and hemodialysis, among other conditions. —Dr. Ryan Huxtable, University of Arizona College of Medicine

---

Revs Up Old Brains: Ginkgo seems to work faster and more efficiently in older people who need it more. According to Italian research, intravenous injections of ginkgo extract increased blood flow in the brain in about 70 percent of subjects. However, younger patients between ages thirty and fifty showed only a 20 percent increase. On the other hand, blood flow jumped 70 percent in those ages fifty to seventy! Also, it took much less time for increased blood flow to peak in the elderly than in the young.

Revives Memory Fast: In some cases, memory improvement can be swift. In a double-blind French study of eighteen elderly men and women, average age sixty-nine, who had a slight memory impairment, ginkgo improved the speed at which they processed information. Researchers gave each subject a massive dose of either 320 or 600 milligrams of ginkgo biloba or a placebo one hour before the test. The ginkgo cut nearly in half the amount of time needed to process the information.

Slows Down Early Alzheimer's: Ginkgo even seems to help alleviate the symptoms of early Alzheimer's disease, according to a first-of-its-kind double-blind German study of forty patients diagnosed with Alzheimer's. Ginkgo in doses of 80 milligrams three times a day caused significant improvements in memory, attention and psychomotor performance after one month. Since Alzheimer's is believed to be partly a result of free radical damage, it's likely that ginkgo's antioxidant activity may help slow down its progression, especially if given early enough. As Dr. Donald J. Brown, director of Natural Product Research Consultants in Seattle, says: "Ginkgo biloba extract may be one of the few 'smart drugs' that actually lives up to its billing."

Improves Peripheral Circulation: As you get older, you may experience leg pain from restricted blood flow to the peripheral arteries, a condition known as intermittent claudication. Pain results when blood circulation is too weak, causing oxygen deprivation of muscles and production of toxins and free radicals. There's firm evidence ginkgo can alleviate this problem by stimulating circulation. A German statistical study, called a meta-analysis, of five trials showed that patients were able to walk much farther during treadmill tests after they had been given ginkgo compared with a placebo.

In one six-month German test, ginkgo stretched the distance patients could walk without pain by more than 100 percent in one-third of the subjects. Distance improved about 30 percent in the other subjects.

THE ANTIAGING PROMISE OF GINKGO

Here's what ginkgo may do, according to current research:

▲ Improve blood flow through arteries, veins and capillaries.

▲ Improve failing memory and information processing in the elderly.

▲ Slow the progression of Alzheimer's disease.

▲ Reduce leg pain from diminishing blood flow to limbs.

▲ Inhibit bacterial activity involved in gum disease.

▲ Relieve vertigo or dizziness.

▲ Reduce ringing in the ears (tinnitus).

▲ Inhibit deteriorating vision due to oxygen deprivation of the retina.

▲ Improve hearing loss related to reduced blood flow.

▲ Lower blood pressure.

▲ Raise good-type HDL cholesterol.

▲ Inhibit abnormal blood clotting.

▲ Relieve male impotence by promoting blood flow to the penis.

▲ Relieve Raynaud's disease, a circulatory disease resulting in cold hands and feet.

What Type and How Much? Nearly all the scientific studies done have used a standardized form of ginkgo called EGb 761, which is made by the German firm of Willmar Schwabe and sold in the United States under the brand name Ginkgold in tablet form. It contains 24 percent of certain compounds called flavone glycosides and is widely available in health food stores. Usual dosage is one standardized 40-milligram ginkgo tablet three times daily to relieve aging problems. Note: You don't get the same benefits from brewing a cup of tea made with leaves from a nearby ginkgo tree.

How Long to See Benefits? On typical doses of 120 milligrams daily, it usually takes at least four to six weeks and sometimes longer to see a benefit from ginkgo. In a recent German study, short-term memory improved after six weeks and learning ability after six months. Ginkgo is not a permanent fix. To maintain benefits, you must continuously take the herb; when you stop, blood flow and other ginkgo-inspired changes return to "normal."

How Much Is Too Much? Ginkgo is considered exceptionally safe among natural drugs. It has caused mild adverse reactions, such as upset stomach and headaches. But severe side effects have not been recorded. One study found that one-half of 1 percent of a group of eighty-five hundred people had mild and reversible side effects, such as stomach upset, while taking ginkgo for up to six months. Moreover, daily doses of 120 milligrams and more have been known to cause transient dizziness initially in some elderly patients. If this happens, reducing the dose may correct it. For therapeutic purposes, one way to overcome initial headaches and dizziness in the elderly, say experts, is to start with a lower dose and gradually increase the dosage over a period of six weeks. This should be done with medical supervision.

Caution: People on any prescription medication or those with blood-clotting disorders should consult their doctors before taking ginkgo. Those who notice any side effects from taking ginkgo should stop taking it and consult their doctors.

ANTIAGING SECRETS OF THE EXPERTS

Ronald Klatz, D.O., age forty
President, American Academy of Anti-Aging Medicine

Dr. Klatz is a founder and head of the academy, dedicated to educating physicians in the clinical practice of antiaging medicine. It is the first such organization to deal with aging as a treatable disease.

Dr. Klatz takes these nutritional supplements every day:

- ▲ Vitamin E—800 IU.
- ▲ Vitamin C—2,000 to 12,000 milligrams.
- ▲ Beta carotene—15 milligrams.
- ▲ Selenium—200 micrograms.
- ▲ Coenzyme Q-10—100 milligrams.
- ▲ Ginkgo biloba extract—80 milligrams.
- ▲ Garlic capsules (Kyolic)—12 capsules.
- ▲ A high-dose multivitamin-mineral preparation without iron or copper.

AN AGING PROPHYLACTIC?

A question: Why wait until you have lost your faculties before using ginkgo? Why not take the herb prophylactically to help prevent free radical damage, the same way vitamin E and C and other antioxidants do? Indeed, new research makes a strong case for that. Whereas the sole focus previously was ginkgo's therapeutic activity, much new research shows ginkgo to be a strong antioxidant with general antiaging powers that may prevent the onset of old-age symptoms.

Belgium researchers discovered that ginkgo actually mimics one of the most powerful internally produced antioxidant defenses, superoxide dismutase—the same stuff that restored youth to fruit flies. Japanese researchers found that myricetin and quercetin, two antioxidants concentrated in ginkgo, suppressed free radical damage to brain cells, helping account for its protection of aging oxygen-starved brain cells. They speculate this antioxidant activity from these two flavonoids suppresses free radical oxidation of brain cells.

Thus, a preventive ginkgo dose of up to 40 to 80 milligrams daily started in middle age might help preserve youthful brain functioning in old age. Dr. Ronald Klatz, age forty, president of the American Academy of Anti-Aging Medicine in Chicago, thinks so. He takes 80 milligrams of ginkgo daily as a "neuroprotective" against brain deterioration in old age. "Hopefully, if I start early enough, I won't have as much degeneration later," he says.

Ginkgo seems particularly good for people who are just beginning to notice declines in mental functions. It might delay such deterioration, postponing or eliminating later institutionalization, say experts.

Ancient Antiaging Star

▲ ▲ ▲

(Why You Need Garlic to Stop Aging)

Garlic is one of nature's antiaging wonder drugs. Take it in food or pills. If you like garlic, eat it raw or cooked, crushed or cut. If you don't like garlic, don't want garlic breath, or reject fresh garlic for other reasons, take garlic supplements.

If you want to live a more vital, longer life, feed your cells that ancient medicinal herb, garlic—revered for nearly five thousand years as a health tonic and virtual cure-all. Science now is beginning to understand why. The bulb is packed with at least four hundred chemicals, including many antioxidants, which give it potent activity in guarding cells from damage and your entire body from premature aging.

Every morning, after we do our yoga, we each take a clove of garlic, chop it up and swallow it whole.
—Sarah L. (age 104) and A. Elizabeth (age 102) Delany in their book *Having Our Say: The Delany Sisters' First 100 Years*

HOW GARLIC WORKS
Garlic is an incredibly complex mixture of chemicals, and scientists are still baffled by which substances have the

most profound effects. But it is known that garlic chemicals have a range of talents—as antibiotics, antiviral agents, cholesterol reducers, anticoagulants, blood pressure reducers, cancer inhibitors, decongestants, anti-inflammatory agents and perhaps protectors of aging brain cells. Laboratory animals fed garlic function better in old age and live longer.

How Garlic Can Fight Aging

Blocks and Stifles Cancer: Garlic may help you escape cancer as you get older. People who eat garlic are less apt to get certain cancers, such as stomach and colon. Older women who ate garlic more than once a week were about half as apt to develop colon cancer as women who never ate garlic, according to a study of forty-two thousand older women in Iowa by University of Minnesota researchers. Studies in China and Italy find that garlic and onion eaters have about half the risk of stomach cancer. Moreover, garlic may act after the fact as a chemotherapeutic agent to arrest cancer. New evidence from Memorial Sloan Kettering Cancer Center in New York finds that garlic compounds actually stifle the growth of cancer cells. In one study, Dr. John Pinto of Sloan Kettering found that human prostate cancer cells grew only one-fourth as fast as expected when exposed to a garlic chemical known as SAMC. The implications are clear, says Dr. Pinto: Garlic may not just save people from getting cancer but prolong their lives after they have it. In animal studies, garlic is a reliable antidote to cancers of virtually all types. It seems to inhibit cancer in all tissues, including breast, liver and colon, says John Milner, garlic researcher at Pennsylvania State University.

Lowers Cholesterol: Only one-half to one whole fresh garlic clove a day, or comparable amounts in supplements, lowers high cholesterol (over 200) an average 23 points or about 9 percent, according to a major review of the evidence by Stephen Warshafsky at New York Medical College in Valhalla, New York. His analysis included tests of a daily 900 milligrams of Kwai garlic powder tablets, a spray dried powder, and 1,000 milligrams of Kyolic water extract. Amazingly, the studies suggest that a couple of cloves of garlic or the equivalent in supplements may be as potent as cholesterol-lowering drugs that are deemed effective if they reduce cholesterol 15 percent. You need to take garlic for over a month to get cholesterol-lowering benefits. A similar British meta-analysis, or statistical analysis, of other data found an average cholesterol reduction of 12 percent from garlic supplements.

German researchers at the University of Munich isolated six chemicals in garlic that lower blood cholesterol much the same way the cholesterol-lowering drug Mevacor does, by blocking the liver's production of cholesterol. The garlic suppressed cholesterol synthesis by about 50 percent in test animals. One of garlic's strongest anticholesterol substances was ajoene, a compound that also helps deter blood clots and is found in both raw and cooked garlic.

Detoxifies Cholesterol: Especially crucial, garlic's antioxidant powers block free radicals from oxidizing bad-type LDL cholesterol, thus crippling its ability to clog arteries. In a study by William Harris at the University of Kansas Medical Center, taking six 100 milligram capsules of garlic powder (Kwai) every day for two weeks reduced oxidation of LDL cholesterol by a remarkable 34 percent. This means that although you have high cholesterol, eating garlic tends to neutralize its artery-clogging dangers.

Further, garlic lowers blood pressure. In one double-blind German study, the equivalent of two garlic cloves daily reduced blood pressure from 171/102 to 152/89 after three months.

Fights Clots: Another critical way garlic fights heart disease is by discouraging formation of dangerous clots or "thinning the blood." Garlic blocks blood platelets from sticking to each other or the walls of arteries, a first step in artery clogging. Eric Block, professor of chemistry at the State University of New York at Albany, has isolated a garlic chemical, ajoene (*ajo* is Spanish for "garlic"), with anticoagulant activity equal or superior to that of garlic. Garlic also revs up the clot-dissolving fibrinolytic system. Three cloves of raw garlic a day improved clot-dissolving activity about 20 percent in a double-blind study of Indian medical students. Cooked garlic seems to have even more antithrombotic activity.

Garlic also fights aging and clogging in peripheral arteries as well as heart arteries. It can relieve intermittent claudication (pains in legs due to a blockage in or narrowing of leg arteries). After taking garlic powder (Kwai; 800 milligrams daily), patients with intermittent claudication were able to walk 50 yards farther without stopping than those on a placebo could. Usually victims can walk only short distances at a time because of cramplike pains in the legs. The improvement occurred after five weeks of garlic treatment, according to German researchers.

Stops Heart Attacks: Even after you have heart disease or a heart attack, eating or taking garlic may help save you. Pioneering garlic researcher and cardiologist Arun Bordia at Tagore Medical College in India says garlic seems to help dissolve blockages in arteries, partially "healing" arteries damaged by atherosclerosis. Dr. Bordia has found that feeding garlic to rabbits with severe atherosclerosis reduced the degree of blockage in their arteries. More remarkably, he documented that eating garlic after a heart attack helped prevent subsequent heart attacks and deaths. In his study of 432 heart attack patients, those who ate two or three fresh garlic cloves—raw or cooked— every day suffered only half as many fatalities after two years as those eating no garlic. The benefits were more impressive after three years. During that time, garlic eaters suffered only one-third as many deaths and non-fatal heart attacks as nongarlic eaters.

Dr. Bordia suggests that since the benefits of garlic increased with time, the most plausible explanation is a shrinkage in blockages of coronary arteries.

Rejuvenates Brain and Immunity: Remarkable new animal research in Japan reveals that eating garlic can restore brain functioning and immune functioning in aged rats, two faculties that typically deteriorate with advancing age. Garlic may even help prevent and reverse

---

GARLIC HEART DRUGS

Garlic compounds have been patented as ACE inhibitors to lower blood pressure. The garlic behaves much like a new class of prescription blood pressure drugs called angiotensin-converting enzyme or so-called ACE inhibitors. Garlic extract has also been found to have "beta blocker" activity by decreasing the strength and frequency of vascular muscle contractions. Beta blockers are well-known heart and blood pressure drugs.

Alzheimer's-like "senility," according to Dr. Hiroshi Saito, professor of pharmaceutical sciences at the University of Tokyo, who has screened dozens of natural and synthetic products in a search for new drug treatments for senile dementia. He documented that garlic extract suppresses destruction of rat brain cells (neurons) and, more startling, even stimulates the branching of new brain neurons. Thus, garlic helps ensure brain cell survival and "leads to neural regeneration," says Dr. Saito, meaning old brains can grow younger.

Indeed, he found that garlic pepped up the brains of aged mice. After eating garlic they did better on learning and memory tests than old mice denied garlic. Garlic-eating mice also produced more antibodies and lymphocytes, white cells that fight infections and cancer.

Grind one pound of garlic, add it to a jar with the juice of twenty-four lemons and leave covered for twenty-four days. After which take one teaspoon at night. —Ukrainian remedy for old age debility

---

Stretches Life: Dr. Saito, one of Japan's foremost researchers in aging, also found that garlic stretched the life span of laboratory mice. He says he started testing garlic because it is a well-known ancient Chinese prescription for senile dementia. The aged garlic extract used in his experiments is sold in the United States as Kyolic.

In other research, allicin, a major garlic compound that gives the herb its odor, also revved up production of two powerful internally produced antioxidant enzymes, catalase and glutathione peroxidase, which have proved to be life extenders in lower forms of life.

THE PROZAC OF THE SUPERMARKET

"I suspect garlic is antistress, antianxiety and acts as a sort of antidepressant like Prozac, although with a much milder effect," says Dr. Gilles Fillion of the Pasteur Institute in France. "Eating garlic may just make you feel better."

Dr. Fillion has found that garlic affects the release of serotonin—a ubiquitous brain chemical involved in regulating a wide spectrum of moods and behavior, including anxiety, depression, pain, aggression, stress, sleep and memory. Higher levels of serotonin and serotonin activity in the brain tend to act as a tranquilizer to calm you down, induce sleep and relieve depression. Dr. Fillion believes garlic helps normalize the serotonin system. A Japanese study of mice once found that garlic extract was 60 percent as effective as Valium in relieving stress.

Garlic's ability to impede the degeneration of the brain and immune system in aged animals is striking and impressive. That doesn't mean garlic can restore youth or completely block the aging process, but it can slow it down. —Dr. Yongxiang Zhang, University of Tokyo

---

What Type? "You can eat garlic raw and cooked. You can take supplements of most any type. All of it should work," says Penn State's Dr. John Milner, who has tested many forms of garlic. Even garlic powder right off the spice shelf has antiaging activity, he says. However, cooking and crushing do change garlic's powers. For example, raw crushed or cut garlic contains lots of allicin, the stuff that

gives garlic its characteristic odor and its strong antibacterial traits. Cooked or deodorized garlic does not contain
significant allicin and thus has little or no antibacterial
and antiviral activity. Raw, chopped garlic is most effective as an antibiotic, says Dr. Eric Block.

What About Garlic Pills? In most aspects (but probably
not all), garlic supplements contain the same antiaging
chemicals as fresh garlic. Such supplements have been
widely tested in animals and humans, especially in Germany, Japan and the United States, and exhibited definite
anticancer and cardiovascular benefits. Garlic pills are the
best-selling over-the-counter drug in Germany. And many
researchers in the United States say they regularly take
garlic supplements as well as eat fresh garlic. The most
thoroughly tested garlic supplements are the Japanese-
made Kyolic and German-made Kwai. The makers of
Kyolic boast that 80 percent of the research on garlic has
been done with their product.

Japanese Kyolic, synonymous with cold-pressed "aged
garlic extract," is an odorless liquid or dried powder, aged
in alcohol and full of sulfur compounds. Some researchers
prefer it because it has a standardized amount of one of
garlic's pharmacologically active chemicals, S-allyicysteine.
Kyolic does not contain allicin.

German Kwai is also a well-tested dried garlic preparation that, unlike Kyolic, reportedly does release allicin and
bases much of its health claims on its allicin potential. It
is coated and dissolves in the intestinal tract, not in the
stomach.

Scientists disagree over precisely which compounds in
garlic are most important, and thus which types of supplements are better. However, in well-designed studies, both
Kwai and Kyolic have lowered blood cholesterol and

blood pressure, and produced antioxidant and anticoagulant effects. If you use garlic supplements, take them with meals, experts advise.

How Much? From half a fresh clove to two or three a day should give your cells a youth-saving injection. In one study, heart attack victims who ate a couple of cloves a day, raw or cooked, cut their odds of dying during the next two years by 66 percent. In supplements, 600 to 900 milligrams of active garlic powder per day has produced documented heart-protective effects. About one and a half cloves of garlic blocked formation of carcinogenic nitrosamines in the stomachs of human volunteers at Penn State.

How Potent? The antiaging potency of garlic depends on the size of the clove and the soil in which it is grown. Garlic grown in selenium-rich earth, for example, is particularly rich in the trace mineral selenium, which enhances the bulb's antiaging powers. Here's a rough guide to equivalent doses found in fresh garlic cloves, powder and pills:

Two or three fresh garlic cloves equal one teaspoon of garlic powder (the stuff you find on the spice rack); four one-gram (1,000 milligrams) powdered garlic tablets, such as Kwai; four gel caps of Kyolic garlic; or one teaspoon of liquid Kyolic garlic.

How Much Is Too Much? Raw garlic in high doses can be toxic; there's little danger in cooked garlic. Eating more than three raw garlic cloves a day has caused diarrhea, gas, bloating and fever. Eating more than 20 grams a day (seven to ten cloves) of garlic has been linked to gastric bleeding. With garlic supplements, don't exceed the manufacturer's recommended doses.

THE ANTIAGING PROMISE OF GARLIC

▲ Revs up immune functions.

▲ Reduces high blood cholesterol, about as much as some prescription drugs do.

▲ Acts as an anticoagulant to thin your blood and discourage dangerous blood clots.

▲ Protects aging brains from mental malfunction, including memory loss, diminished thinking and learning abilities, depression, possibly dementia.

▲ Inhibits cell changes leading to cancer and helps destroy cancer cells.

▲ Suppresses general bodily deterioration stemming from free radical attacks on cells.

Garlic contains at least a dozen antioxidants.

A Plateful of Miracles

▲ ▲ ▲

(Why You Must Eat Fruits and
Vegetables to Stop Aging)

Eat all the various fruits and vegetables you can. There is nowhere—repeat, nowhere—you can get the injections of antiaging potions you get from eating fruits and vegetables. They are not trivial creations of nature, but mighty forces to be reckoned with. They possess countless known and unknown agents that transform your cells into fortresses against the free radical forces of aging. Much of what we call aging is really a fruit and vegetable deficiency!

Here's the deal: If you are convinced, as many scientists are, that the main cause of getting old and infirm and dying is an increasing inability of your cells to resist destructive oxygen free radicals, it's logical that the more antioxidants of varying types you get to your cells up to a point, the less rapidly you will succumb to the ravages of aging. There is only one place you find these treasure chests of antioxidants in all their power and glory. That is in fruits and vegetables. "That's where the gold is," says biochemist Bruce Ames. And although it may not sound very exciting, it is. The fruits and vegetables you put in your mouth have magnificent powers to transform the lives of your cells and your destiny, at all times of life, especially as you grow older.

Fruits and vegetables of all kinds are packed with so

many known and unknown antioxidants, it makes the head spin, and it's quite unclear which ones are most powerful. Most experts think many constituents in fruits and vegetables collaborate to combat the ravages of aging. It's unlikely single compounds will emerge as magic bullets, although scientists predict that one day they may be able to extract and synthesize certain components of fruits and vegetables to fight specific diseases and help keep you young. Still, it seems impossible that science will ever perfect a broccoli pill comparable to the real thing. The only sure way to get the total antiaging bounty of nature is to eat fruits and vegetables in their whole, complex, original form.

THE ALARMING FACTS

- More than half of Americans do not eat a single serving of fruit, vegetables or fruit juice on any given day.
- Less than 10 percent of Americans eat five or more servings of fruits and vegetables a day. Most Americans do not even come close.
- Skimping on fruits and vegetables doubles your chances of cancer.

HOW FRUITS AND VEGETABLES FIGHT AGING

The astonishing powers of fruits and vegetables to help stem free radical damage that brings on aging and chronic diseases have been widely documented. Here's how they can help prevent premature aging.

Block Cancer: Incredible as it may seem, eating fruits and vegetables regularly can slash your chances of getting cancer in half! That's the conclusion of an extensive and unimpeachable analysis of nearly two hundred studies from seventeen countries by Gladys Block, Ph.D., cancer researcher at the University of California at Berkeley. Even smokers can partially reverse the damage leading to cancer by eating fruits and vegetables, particularly ones rich in beta carotene (carrots, sweet potatoes, spinach and green leafy vegetables). Eating a mere carrot or half a cup of spinach a day may cut lung cancer risk 50 percent, several studies suggest, even in previously longtime heavy smokers.

Cabbage, broccoli, cauliflower and other cruciferous vegetables contain chemicals that speed the removal of harmful estrogen from the body, thwarting breast cancer. Tomato eaters are five times less likely to develop pancreatic cancer, Johns Hopkins investigators found.

Women eating the most fruits and vegetables, particularly deep orange and green vegetables, had about half the risk of endometrial cancer as women who ate the least, a Swiss study found. A University of Alabama study also singled out beta carotene–rich vegetables as a major deterrent to endometrial cancer.

Even after cancer is diagnosed, eating lots of vegetables and fruits can hinder the progression of cancer. Scientists at the Cancer Research Center in Hawaii studied the diets of 463 men and 212 women with lung cancer. Women who loaded up on vegetables nearly doubled their survival time compared with those eating the least vegetables. Among men, tomatoes, oranges and broccoli appeared to improve survival chances.

It's never too late to lower your risk of a future cardiovascular event by eating more fruits and vegetables. —Dr. JoAnn Manson, assistant professor of medicine at Harvard Medical School

---

ANTIAGING SECRETS OF THE EXPERTS

Walter Willett, M.D.
Professor of Epidemiology and Nutrition,
Harvard University School of Public Health

Dr. Willett is the author of numerous studies finding that diet and antioxidants greatly influence susceptibility to chronic diseases, such as heart disease and cancer. He takes these supplements daily:

▲ Vitamin E—400 IU.
▲ Multivitamin-mineral tablet (mostly for folate and B vitamins).

"The dosage is safe, the cost minimal. So why not cover the bases?" He eats no meat or margarine, and follows a Mediterranean diet, plentiful in olive oil, fruits and vegetables.

Prevent Cardiovascular Disease: Eating lots of fruits and vegetables can save you from heart attacks and strokes and even help "unclog" arteries after heart attacks, much research shows. A recent Harvard study found that women who ate an additional carrot or other high-carotene food daily slashed their risk of heart attack by 22 percent and stroke by as much as 70 percent. Other research shows that stroke victims with high blood levels of fruit and vegetable carotenoids are less likely to die or have permanent damage. A diet rich in fruits and vegetables also helps curb high blood pressure. In an Italian study, 81 percent of those who began eating three to six servings of fruits and vegetables daily were able to cut their doses of blood pressure medication in half. Some no longer needed drugs at all.

Preserve Mental and Physical Faculties: It's mind-boggling to think that a deficiency of a tomato chemical could impair your ability to cope in old age. But Dr. David Snowdon and colleagues at the University of Kentucky have found that true in their studies of elderly women. Those with the lowest blood levels of a red pigment called lycopene, an antioxidant, scored lowest in mental and physical functioning. Virtually the only way lycopene gets in your blood is if you eat tomatoes. (It's also in watermelon and to a slight degree in apricots.)

In Dr. Snowdon's study of eighty-eight women over age seventy-five, those with low blood lycopene were less able to perform "self care tasks," such as walking, bathing, dressing, feeding and toileting. In fact, women low in lycopene were four times more apt to require assistance than those with above-average lycopene. Dr. Snowdon theorizes that over the years a lycopene deficiency allowed free radicals to damage joints, muscles and brain cells, leading to a decline in general overall physical and mental functions. "Low lycopene marks mental and physical disability," concludes Dr. Snowdon.

A lack of folic acid, concentrated in green leafy vegetables as well as legumes, is also associated with failing mental faculties and depression.

Save Eyesight: People who eat less than three and a half servings of fruits and vegetables a day are four times more prone to cataracts as they get older, according to research by Paul Jacques at Tufts University. In particular, carotenoids, vitamin C and folic acid, rich in fruits and vegetables, seem to combat free radical damage that cause the opacity of the lens known as cataract. Spinach seems to have special vision-protecting powers. A recent study in the *British Medical Journal* identified spinach as the food most apt to prevent cataracts in a group of elderly women. Spinach is also likely to save you from another vision-destroying disease of aging, macular degeneration that results from years of free radical damage to the tiny central part of the retina, called the macula. Johanna M. Seddon, an ophthalmologist at the Massachusetts Eye and Ear Infirmary, finds that people eating the most carotenoid-rich vegetables, such as spinach, collard greens and kale, slashed their odds of macular degeneration by 43 percent compared with those eating the least.

How to Put Aging on Hold

- ▲ Eat at least five to nine servings of fruits and vegetables a day. A serving is one-half cup cooked or chopped raw fruit or vegetables; one cup of raw leafy vegetables; one medium piece of fruit or six ounces of fruit juice or vegetable juice.
- ▲ Eat lots of different fruits and vegetables because scientists don't yet know which might be the most powerfully protective.
- ▲ Choose fresh and frozen fruits and vegetables over canned ones when possible. Although canning does not destroy all types of antioxidants, it does destroy some, in particular, glutathione and indoles.
- ▲ Eat both whole fruits and vegetables and juices. Juice, extracted from fruits and vegetables, contains antiaging substances, but not the entire spectrum found in the whole fruit or vegetable.

However, you can buy high-powered blenders that crush the entire fruit or vegetable, retaining everything, including the seeds and membranes in citrus fruits, for example. In that case, you get even more from the liquefied version than from the intact food if you like drinking your fruits and vegetables.

▲ Eat vegetables both raw and lightly cooked; both ways have advantages. Raw foods generally are highest in antioxidants; cooking destroys some, but not others. In fact, light cooking boosts absorption of beta carotene. Eat vegetables such as broccoli and cauliflower raw or cook them only until still crunchy (al dente), since heavy cooking destroys critical antiaging components.

▲ To get the most antioxidants, choose deeply colored fruits and vegetables. The deep pigment is often a giveaway for antioxidants. For example, the darkest orange carrots and sweet potatoes and the deepest green leafy vegetables, such as spinach and lettuces, contain the most antioxidant carotenoids, including beta carotene and lutein. Red grapes, red onions and yellow onions have much more antioxidant quercetin than green grapes and white onions. Blueberries, because of their deep hues, contain exceptionally high concentrations of antioxidant flavonoids.

▲ To retain the most antioxidants in cooked vegetables, microwave them. For example, microwaving broccoli destroyed only 15 percent of vitamin C whereas boiling in half a cup of water destroyed about 50 percent, according to U.S. Department of Agriculture tests. Steaming, grilling and stir-frying vegetables also generally preserve more antioxidants than heavy boiling.

TEN SUPER-ANTIAGING FRUITS
AND VEGETABLES

Any fruit or vegetable you eat is bound to make known and unknown chemical contributions to your quest for youth. But here are ten with so much known potential you shouldn't ignore them.

Note: Garlic is a super-antiaging food that you can also take in pill form. (See page 158.)

1. AVOCADO: It's one of the super-guardians of cells because of its abundance of glutathione, the "master antioxidant" that, among other miracles, helps neutralize highly destructive fat in foods (see page 128). True, avocado is high-fat, but much of it is good fat—monounsaturated, a type that resists oxidation. Eating avocados also lowers and improves blood cholesterol, better than a low-fat diet does, according to recent research. The fruit is also rich in blood-vessel protective potassium.

2. BERRIES: Blueberries, cranberries, strawberries, raspberries—they are all loaded with antioxidants to save your cells from premature aging. Blueberries, for example, have more antioxidants called anthocyanins than any other food—three times more than the second richest sources, red wine and green tea. Both blueberries and cranberries help ward off urinary tract infections. In one study, older people who ate the most strawberries had the lowest rate of all kinds of cancer. Berries are particularly rich in antioxidant vitamin C, an overall youth potion.

3. BROCCOLI: It's hard to say enough for the antiaging properties of broccoli. It is blessed with an awesome array of antioxidants. Particularly strong is one called sulforaphane, discovered by Johns Hopkins scientists. Fed to animals, the broccoli chemical revved up the activity of detoxification enzymes that slashed cancer rate by two-thirds. Broccoli is packed with free radical fighters vitamin C, beta carotene, quercetin, indoles, glutathione and lutein. Broccoli is one of the richest food sources of the trace metal chromium, a life extender and protector against the ravages of out-of-control insulin and blood sugar. In women, broccoli helps the body get rid of the harmful type of estrogen that promotes cancer. Broccoli eaters also have less colon and lung cancer and cardiovascular disease. Eating broccoli has even been linked to longer survival in lung cancer patients.

4. CABBAGE: Like broccoli, cabbage is a cruciferous vegetable with potent antioxidant activity. Men who ate cabbage once a week compared with once a month had only 66 percent the risk of colon cancer, one classic study found. Cabbage also seems to deter stomach and breast cancer. A specific antioxidant in cabbage, indole-3-carbinol, accelerates the disposal of a harmful form of estrogen that promotes breast cancer. Dr. H. Leon Bradlow, at the Strang Cornell Cancer Research Laboratory in New York City, found that about 70 percent of a large group of women who ate cabbage started burning off dangerous estrogen within five days. Effective dose is a fifth to a third of a head of cabbage. Savoy cabbage (the crinkly type) is strongest. To get the most antiaging benefits, eat cabbage and other cruciferous vegetables raw or lightly cooked.

5. CARROTS: Carrots are legendary in fighting off aging diseases. A recent Harvard study found that women who ate carrots at least five times a week reduced their risk of having a stroke by 68 percent! In other research, eating a couple of carrots a day lowered blood cholesterol by 10 percent in men. Countless studies pinpoint beta carotene, carrots' main antioxidant asset, as a powerhouse against aging and disease. The beta carotene in a daily medium carrot cuts lung cancer risk in half, even among former heavy smokers. People with low levels of beta carotene in their blood are more apt to have heart attacks and various cancers and to die or be disabled by strokes. Beta carotene helps protect the eyes from sight-robbing diseases that develop with aging. The orange pigment also boosts immune functioning. One medium carrot contains about 6 milligrams of beta carotene. For a real injection of beta carotene, try carrot juice. One cup contains 24 milligrams of beta carotene.

6. CITRUS FRUIT: The orange is so full of antioxidants that officials at the National Cancer Institute have called it a complete package of every class of natural anticancer inhibitor known, including carotenoids, terpenes, flavonoids, and vitamin C. Grapefruit, too, has a unique type fiber, especially in the membranes and juice sacs, that reduces cholesterol dramatically and even may reverse the aging disease atherosclerosis. Grapefruit is also high in glutathione, the so-called master antioxidant that fights off all kinds of free radical damage to cells—and thus aging.

7. GRAPES: The antiaging secret of grapes is simple and powerful: Grapes contain twenty known antioxidants that work together to fend off oxygen free radical attacks that promote disease and aging, according to researchers at the University of California, Davis. The antioxidants are in the skin and seeds, and the more colorful the skin, the greater the antioxidant punch. That means red and purple grapes and purple grape juice are more powerful. Grape antioxidants have anticlogging activity, inhibit oxidation of LDL cholesterol and relax blood vessels. Indeed, tests at the University of Wisconsin find that three glasses of purple grape juice and one glass of red wine have equal anticlotting effects in arteries. The antioxidant quercetin, also plentiful in onions and tea, appears to be one of grapes' foremost antiaging components.

Raisins, which are simply dried grapes, count too. In fact, raisins contain higher concentrations of antiaging compounds than fresh grapes—but not as much as red wine, according to tests by Gene Spiller, Ph.D., of the Health Research and Studies Center, Inc., in Los Altos, California. He found raisins have three to five times more of certain phenols or antioxidants as fresh grapes. A serving of raisins (one and a half ounces) also had three times more of the antioxidants than a glass of white wine, and one-third as much of the antioxidants as a glass of typical French red wine.

8. ONIONS: A close kin of garlic, the onion, too, has diverse antiaging activity. Full of antioxidants, onions help prevent cancer, especially stomach cancer, "thin the blood," discouraging clots, and raise good-type HDL cholesterol. Red and yellow onions (not white onions) are the richest foods in quercetin, a celebrated antioxidant that inactivates cancer-causing agents, inhibits enzymes that spur cancer growth, has anti-inflammatory, antibacterial, antifungal and antiviral activity. Quercetin also keeps bad LDL cholesterol from turning toxic and attacking arteries. In studies, onions have quashed the ability of fats, such as butter, to initiate formation of blood clots to clog arteries. In horses, onions have long been used to dissolve blood clots.

9. SPINACH: This green leafy vegetable is packed with a variety of antioxidants. No wonder spinach and its components often show up in studies as warding off a broad variety of free radical–inspired diseases, including cancer, heart disease, high blood pressure, strokes, cataracts, macular degeneration, even psychiatric problems. One of the most striking antioxidants in spinach is lutein, thought to be as strong an antiaging agent as well-known beta carotene. Spinach, however, is rich in both. Eating high amounts of spinach cuts the risk of macular degeneration, a potential cause of blindness, by 45 percent. Eating a cup of raw spinach or a half cup of cooked spinach daily may slash lung cancer odds in half, even among former heavy smokers. Spinach is very rich in folic acid—a brain and artery protector—as well as an anticancer agent.

10. TOMATOES: The familiar tomato is an unexpected antiaging powerhouse. Tomatoes are by far the richest and virtually only reliable source of a remarkable antioxidant, lycopene. German tests show lycopene more powerful in snuffing out specific free radicals than even much-touted beta carotene. Mind-boggling new research suggests that lycopene preserves mental and physical functioning among the elderly. High blood levels of lycopene also reduce your risk of pancreatic and cervical cancer. In new Italian research, those who downed the most raw tomatoes were also only half as likely to have cancers of the digestive tract—oral cavity, pharynx, esophagus, stomach, colon or rectum—as those eating the least tomatoes. Tomato chemicals—p-coumaric acid and chlorogenic acid—suppress formation of cancer-causing nitrosamines. Only tomatoes and watermelon contain substantial amounts of lycopene. Apricots have a smidgen. Cooking and canning tomatoes do not destroy lycopene. That makes tomato juice, canned tomatoes and all kinds of tomato sauces a potent preserver of youth.

VEGETARIANS LIVE LONGER

For sure, eating more fruits and vegetables and less meat can blunt the consequences of aging and prolong your life. But eating only plant foods (and seafood) seems to give you the best odds on aging slowly and stretching your life to the maximum. Vegetarians weigh less, have lower cholesterol and blood pressure, experience fewer heart attacks and cancers, have stronger immune systems and simply outlive meat eaters.

Vegetarians are 28 percent less apt to die of heart disease and 39 percent less likely to die of cancer than meat eaters, according to a 1994 study of six thousand vegetarians by British scientists at the London School of Hygiene and Tropical Medicine.

Even vegetarians who smoked and were obese were less apt to die than smoking, obese meat eaters.

Among Seventh Day Adventists, according to a large-scale study of 27,530 persons, death rates climbed along with the increased consumption of meat and poultry. Striking was the fact that among men, those who had become vegetarians at an early age were less apt to die of heart disease. Similarly, researchers at the University of North Carolina found that the fruits, so to speak, of being a vegetarian in your youth may not become evident until adulthood.

If we—that is, society—switched to a vegetarian diet, atherosclerotic coronary artery disease which accounts for most heart disease would vanish.
—William Roberts, M.D., editor-in-chief of the *American Journal of Cardiology*

Women vegetarians seem to be spared cancers of the breast and ovaries. Meat-eating women consistently have higher circulating levels of estrogen than vegetarian women, probably due to eating more saturated animal fats, studies have found. Estrogen promotes breast and ovarian cancer. Vegetarians also have less colon cancer.

Further, vegetarians have less Type II diabetes, gallstones, kidney stones, osteoporosis and arthritis.

One secret of vegetarians, making them less susceptible to aging and disease in general, is a more vigorous immune system.

A recent German study of male vegetarians documented that their white cells were twice as lethal to tumor cells as those of meat eaters. In fact, vegetarians needed only half as many white cells to do the same job as carnivores did. Their white cells just seemed to be more ferocious.

Question: Do vegetarians live longer and stay younger and healthier because they eat lots of vegetables or because they avoid meat? It's probably both, say experts. They avoid the pro-aging stuff in meat and get the benefits of the antiaging stuff in fruits and vegetables.

WHY VEGETARIANS AGE MORE SLOWLY

They have much higher levels of plant antioxidants in their bloodstreams that ward off aging and chronic diseases.

They have more feisty immune systems to ward off infections and other immune-related diseases, including cancer.

They take in lower levels of iron, concentrated in meat, that encourages cell-destroying free radical activity.

They generally eat fewer calories and lower amounts of dangerous fats.

Magic Marine Oil for Your Cells

▲   ▲   ▲

(Why You Need to Eat Fish to Stop Aging)

Eat at least two or three servings of fish a week, preferably fatty fish, to protect cells against aging attacks. Fish is the one food in which less fat is not better!

One reason you may be aging faster than need be: You don't eat enough seafood. Thus, your cells are left deficient in fish oil. Without enough of this unique pharmacological fat, your cells go bonkers and issue all kinds of inappropriate chemical messages that wreck your joints, clog your arteries, produce pain and spur cancer growth—in other words, accelerate your bodily destruction and demise. No question, fish eaters are more apt to escape aging diseases, such as heart disease, cancer, arthritis, diabetes, psoriasis and bronchitis, studies consistently show. And fish eaters around the world live longer. The Japanese, who hold the world's record for longevity, eat three times more fish than Americans.

All seafood, but fatty fish in particular, such as salmon, tuna, mackerel and sardines, are rich in a peculiar type of fat, called omega-3 fatty acids. This oil mainly protects arteries by "thinning the blood," somewhat as aspirin does, thus discouraging blood clotting that triggers heart attacks and strokes. Such marine fat also lowers blood pressure and triglycerides, a potentially dangerous blood fat, raises good-type HDL cholesterol, regulates heart-beats, makes aged arteries more flexible and helps block inflammatory processes that promote arthritis, cancer, psoriasis, diabetes and general cell dysfunction. Seafood is also rich in powerful antioxidants, including selenium and ubiquinol (coenzyme Q-10), that fight disease and general aging. Salmon, mackerel and sardines are especially high in coenzyme Q-10.

How Fish Can Fight Aging

Extends Life: You can defy death and add years to your life by taking up fish eating, even if you have already been felled by heart disease. In a famous British study, William Burr, M.D., at the Medical Research Council in Cardiff, Wales, told victims of heart attacks either to eat more oily fish, such as salmon and sardines—at least two servings a week—or to eat more fiber or to eat less fat. During the next two years, the death rates among the fish eaters dropped about 30 percent. There was no reduction of heart disease or extension of life from cutting down on fat or eating more fiber.

Keeps Arteries Young: The more fish oil in body cells, the less clogged and aged the arteries, Danish investigators found during random autopsies. Also, fish eaters (more than eight ounces a week) were only half as likely to have their arteries close up again after angioplasty (a procedure to dilate arteries) than non–fish eaters, Canadian researchers found. Most effective were fatty fish, such as salmon and sardines. On the other hand, a major study found that taking fish oil capsules did not tend to keep arteries open after angioplasty.

Fish oil is one of the most reliable ways of slashing

triglycerides, a dangerous blood fat. In studies, taking fish oil or eating salmon also raises good-type HDL cholesterol.

Cuts Heart Attacks: Averaging a mere ounce of fish a day cuts your chances of having a heart attack in half, a landmark Dutch study found. A newly discovered way fish oil fights heart attacks is by directly improving heart function, helping block arrhythmias and ventricular fibrillation, irregular heartbeats that can trigger sudden death. In Australian studies, feeding monkeys even very small amounts of fish oil saved them from developing fatal heart arrhythmias. Similarly, Ohio State University research on monkeys documented that fish oil infusions blocked potentially fatal fibrillation following a heart attack 87 percent of the time.

Restores Artery Elasticity: Taking 3,000 milligrams of fish oil a day (the amount in seven ounces of mackerel or canned sardines) made stiffened, aged arteries significantly more flexible, allowing them to stretch better in response to changes in blood pressure, University of Minnesota researchers found.

Wards Off Diabetes: Eating a mere one ounce of fish a day of any kind—lean, fatty or canned—compared with eating no fish, cut the odds of developing Type II diabetes in half, theoretically by helping prevent glucose intolerance, government researchers in the Netherlands reported.

Curtails Strokes: Men who ate at least five ounces of fish a week had half the risk of stroke as non–fish eaters, probably because of thinner blood and fewer blood clots, according to a recent Dutch study.

Thwarts Colon Cancer: A major Italian study showed that daily doses of fish oil (comparable to that in eight ounces of mackerel) suppressed abnormal cell growth by 62 percent in 90 percent of those vulnerable to colon cancer. And researchers observed the slowdown in only two weeks' time!

Blocks Breast Cancer: Fish oil seems to retard the spread—or metastasis—of breast cancer, say Harvard researchers. Breast cancer is five times lower in Japan, where women eat the most fish. A recent Belgian study of breast cancer death rates in thirty countries showed that fish eaters had lower rates than non–fish eaters. Highest death rates were for women eating animal fat. Further, studies by David P. Rose, Ph.D., at the American Health Foundation, a major nonprofit health research organization, found that mice on a high fish oil diet were only 40 percent as likely to have tumors that metastasized or spread as those fed a diet high in corn oil.

Protects Smokers' Lungs: Eating fish can even block some of the tremendous free radical burden of cigarette smoking by slowing deterioration of lung function. In one study of nearly nine thousand current or former smokers, those who averaged four fish servings per week were 45 percent less apt to have bronchitis or emphysema than those eating one-half fish serving or less per week. Theory: Fish oil inhibits inflammatory reactions leading to cell damage.

How Does Fish Work?

Much of fish's benefits are attributed to its high content of a unique type fat called omega-3 fatty acids. Among other things, these omega-3s help discourage formation of hormonelike agents called prostaglandins that can trigger inflammatory processes destroying arteries and joints and encouraging cancer and overall cell malfunction. One way the omega-3s do this is by replacing excessive amounts of the terrible omega-6 fatty acids, fats predominant in corn and sunflower seed oils, that are readily oxidized factories for free radicals.

In short, if you have too much omega-6 and too little omega-3, as most Americans do, the omega-6s overwhelm and dominate activity in cells, causing much destruction. Many experts think aging diseases run rampant because we typically eat ten times more destructive omega-6s in fats than omega-3s. Anything you do to right this imbalance helps preserve your youth. Animal studies also show that omega-3 fatty acids help rev up antioxidant enzyme activity and omega-6 oils turn it down.

Fish oil consistently decreases the size of tumors in animals, the number of tumors and their tendency to spread, which is exactly the opposite of what corn oil does. —Dr. Artemis Simopoulos, president of the Center for Genetics, Nutrition and Health in Washington, D.C.

How to Get Antiaging Fish Oil

▲ Eat fatty fish. Fish with the most antiaging omega-3 are mackerel, anchovies, fresh and canned herring, fresh and canned salmon, canned sardines, fresh tuna and sablefish. Fish with moderate amounts are turbot, shark, bluefish, canned albacore (white) tuna, striped bass, smelt, oysters, swordfish, bass, rainbow trout and pompano.

▲ Eat sardines canned in water or in their own omega-3 rich–oil labeled "sild oil."

▲ Eat fish without lots of added fat, such as mayonnaise, butter and cream sauces. Such foods tend to overwhelm your cells with bad fat, leading to much cell damage and canceling out some of the antiaging effects of fish. Deep-frying also negates antiaging properties.

▲ Particularly avoid eating omega-6 fatty acids, as in corn oil, regular safflower and sunflower oils. These are most apt to neutralize fish powers in cells by spewing off lots of free radicals that can damage cells.

Can You Get Too Much? Be aware that eating lots of oily fish tends to prolong bleeding time and may lower immunity. Don't overdose on fatty fish or fish oil capsules if you are on anticoagulants or any blood thinning drugs. Consult your physician. If you eat fish every day, you should be sure to take vitamin E capsules (200 to 400 IU daily) to preserve optimum immune functioning, according to research by Simin Meydani, Tufts University.

What About Fish Oil Capsules? Dr. Alexander Leaf, emeritus professor of preventive medicine at Harvard University School of Public Health, prefers you eat fish, but he also says it's okay to take up to a gram (1,000 milligrams) of omega-3 fish oil daily in capsules. You usually get that amount in three capsules of a brand such as MaxEpa. If you take fish oil capsules, be sure to take vitamin E to keep immune functioning up to par. Take high therapeutic doses of fish oil only with medical supervision.

FISH OIL WITHOUT THE FISH

You can also get lifesaving, antiaging omega-3s in certain plant foods. Exceptionally high in terrestrial omega-3s are wheat germ oil, canola oil, walnuts and soybeans, purslane (a wild green carried in some health food markets) and flaxseed oil.

The plant omega-3s are an alternative, especially if you are a vegetarian, but they are less biologically active than omega-3s in fish oil.

OMEGA-3 FATTY ACIDS IN PLANTS

High	Grams of Omega-3 Per 100 Grams ($3^1/2$ Ounces)
Wheat germ oil	6.9
Butternuts	8.7
Walnut oil	10.4
Canola oil	11.1
Flaxseed oil	53.3

Medium	
Purslane	0.9
Oat germ	1.4
Beechnuts	1.7
Soybeans, kernels, roasted	1.5
Soybeans, green	3.2
Soybean oil	6.8
Walnuts, Persian English	6.8

Source: U.S. Department of Agriculture

Asian Secret to Long Life

▲   ▲   ▲

(Why You Need Soybeans to Stop Aging)

If you don't eat soybeans, you deprive yourself of a readily available youth potion. One of the best things you can do to enliven your cells' defenses against aging and age-related diseases is to infuse them with substances found in the soybean.

The soybean may seem like a tiny speck of nature, a trivial, inconsequential creation. Wrong. It is actually an antiaging pill, packed with powerful antioxidants that can perform magic in your cells. Inside your body the soybean is a mighty force that may actually alter your destiny, slowing the pace with which you age and consequently influencing when you encounter disease and death.

That's what Dr. Denham Harman, the father of the free radical theory of aging, discovered a couple of decades ago. He found that soybeans could interfere with free radical damage, which is at the heart of how fast you age. Laboratory animals fed soybean protein had far less free radical damage to their cells than animals fed casein, a protein in milk and other dairy products. In short, eating soybeans slowed down aging; eating milk or animal protein accelerated it. Eating soybeans instead of casein also stretched the animals' life spans by 13 percent!

This may help illuminate why vegetarians enjoy a longer life and why the Japanese, who eat the most soybeans in the world—thirty times more than Americans—live longer than anyone.

Recently, scientists have identified the source of the soybean's enormous biochemical energy. The bean is a powerhouse of antioxidants and other antidisease agents, including genistein, daidzein, protease inhibitors, phytates, saponins, phytosterols, phenolic acids and lecithin. Many are antioxidants, able to battle aging and chronic diseases on many fronts. For example, Dr. Ann R. Kennedy, University of Pennsylvania School of Medicine, finds that a protease inhibitor in soybeans—called Bowman-Birk inhibitor—is so versatile against various cancers that she calls it "a universal cancer preventive agent." Dr. Stephen Barnes, professor of pharmacology at the University of Alabama at Birmingham, hails soy's genistein as a unique and incredibly promising inhibitor of breast and prostate cancer. Dr. Harman also points out that the amino acids in soybeans are less vulnerable to oxidation; thus, unlike many other foods, soybeans don't spew scads of damaging free radicals throughout your body to mangle and age your cells.

THE DRUG THAT MAKES SOYBEANS SPECIAL

Soybeans are unique because they are a rare source of high concentrations of a kind of wonder drug, known as genistein. Genistein is a potent antioxidant with wide-ranging biological antiaging and anticancer activity. For example, genistein interferes with fundamental cancer processes at virtually every stage: Genistein blocks an enzyme that turns on cancer genes, thwarting cancer at inception. It inhibits angiogenesis, the spawning of new blood vessels needed to feed growing cancers. In test tubes, it directly curbs the growth of all types of cancer cells—of the breast, colon, lung, prostate, skin and blood (leukemia). It also has antihormonal effects that give it special potential in deterring breast and possibly prostate cancer.

On other antiaging fronts, genistein saves arteries because, just as it hinders cancer cell proliferation, it also obstructs proliferation of smooth muscle cells in artery walls that promotes plaque buildup and clogged arteries. And genistein clamps down on the activity of an enzyme, thrombin, that promotes blood clotting, thus heart attacks and strokes. Remarkably, genistein also seems to actually decrease the number of cells that are dividing in the breast. This gives enzymes more time to repair DNA damage so it is not permanently passed on to newly created cells in the form of mutations that hasten aging and cancer.

Even more astonishing, a brief exposure to soybean genistein early in life may inoculate against cancer. Investigations at the University of Alabama by Dr. Barnes's colleague Coral Lamartiniere have found that even very low doses of genistein given soon after birth to female rats delays the onset, size and multiplicity of cancers in middle and old age. In the experiment, a group of newborn rats were given a chemical known to cause breast cancer later in life. Some also were given genistein and others got an inactive compound. Of those getting genistein at birth, only 60 percent developed breast cancer in mid to late life. One hundred percent of those getting the dummy pill developed tumors. This might mean infants now drinking soy-based formula or who drank it thirty years ago have already received a dose of anticancer vaccine, partially immunizing them against future malignancies, Dr. Barnes says, but as yet no human studies have been done to verify it.

So powerful is genistein that researchers see it as a potential new type anticancer drug. But why wait? You can get the drug now by eating soybeans.

Another soybean compound, daidzein, has some but not all genistein's powers. Daidzein, too, blocks cancer in animals and is also an isoflavone with antiestrogenic activity. These two soy compounds—genistein plus daidzein—are considered double threats to rapid aging and cancer in particular.

THE ALARMING FACTS

▲ We grow about half the world's soybeans and export one-third of it, mainly to Japan. Nearly all that we keep goes into food for pets and agricultural animals.

▲ The Japanese, who hold the world's record for longevity, eat about an ounce of soy per day. Americans eat too little to measure. Americans have four times more fatal breast cancer and five times more prostate cancer than the Japanese.

HOW SOYBEANS CAN FIGHT AGING

Prevents Breast Cancer: You may be more vulnerable to breast cancer not because of the fat you eat, but because of the soybeans you don't eat, says Dr. Barnes. His studies show that giving soybeans or soy's essential chemical genistein to animals slashes breast cancer rates by 40 to 65 percent. Japanese women, who regularly eat soybean foods, have only one-fourth as much breast cancer as American women. A recent study found that premenopausal women in Singapore who ate the most soy protein foods had only half as much breast cancer as average soy protein consumers.

ANTIAGING SECRETS OF THE EXPERTS

Andrew Weil, M.D.
University of Arizona College of Medicine

Dr. Weil is one of the most highly respected practitioners of "alternative" medicine, favoring natural substances and antioxidants for the prevention and treatment of disease and aging.

Here's what Dr. Weil takes every day and recommends to others as a "good, safe, daily formula":

▲ Beta carotene—25,000 IU (15 milligrams).
▲ Vitamin E (natural)—400 IU if under age forty or 800 IU if over age forty.
▲ Selenium— 200 micrograms.
▲ Vitamin C—1,000 to 2,000 milligrams, twice a day.

Soybean chemicals seem to combat breast cancer at least two ways: They have a direct anticancer effect on cells. They also manipulate estrogen much the way the cancer-fighting drug tamoxifen does—by blocking estrogen's ability to stimulate malignant changes in breast tissue. Thus, soybeans should help thwart the occurrence and spread of breast cancer in both premenopausal and postmenopausal women.

Blocks Prostate Cancer: Soybeans may also explain the mystery of why Japanese men develop prostate cancer, but don't die of it at the rate Western men do. Indeed, Japanese men are just as prone to small, latent prostate cancers as Westerners. But, in the Japanese, the cancers don't grow fast enough to become deadly. It's the soybeans, insists Finnish researcher Herman Adlercreutz. In one study, he found up to 110 times more soybean chemicals in the blood of Japanese men than in the blood of Finnish men. It's well-known, he says, that eating soy products dramatically curbs prostate cancer in laboratory animals. Moreover, the soybean constituent genistein can actually block the spread of prostate cancer cells in test-tube experiments. Dr. Adlercreutz theorizes that soybean chemicals exert an antihormonal effect that impedes the growth of prostate cancer cells so they do not form potentially deadly tumors.

Your risk of cancer doubles if you don't eat soybeans regularly. —Dr. Mark Messina, coauthor of *The Simple Soybean and Your Health*

Saves Arteries: Soybeans are antidotes to old arteries. Soybean protein itself actually discourages and may help reverse arterial disease. Extensive research by Italian investigators at the University of Milan found that eating soybean protein instead of meat and dairy protein caused high blood cholesterol to plunge as much as 21 percent in three weeks. The soybeans worked even when subjects were on high-cholesterol diets. Moreover, soy boosted good-type HDL cholesterol about 15 percent and depressed triglycerides. Doctors also documented that blood flow to the heart had improved, suggesting a rejuvenation of arteries.

Further, soy milk, like vitamin E, blocks the oxidation

of bad LDL cholesterol, thus preventing it from harming arteries, according to new Japanese research.

Regulates Blood Sugar: You can count on soybeans to combat treacherous insulin in your blood and keep blood sugar levels on an even keel, thus slowing down the progression toward diabetes and heart disease. In particular, soybeans are rich in two amino acids, glycine and arginine, that reduce insulin. In studies by Dr. David Jenkins of the University of Toronto, soybeans proved second only to peanuts in promoting a desirable flat blood sugar response and thus lower insulin. High blood insulin and blood sugar are incriminated in cell destruction and aging. (See page 281.)

Builds Stronger Bones: Eating lots of soy protein, such as soy milk, soybeans and tofu, as Asian women do, helps build strong bones, according to Mark Messina, Ph.D., formerly at the National Cancer Institute and now a food science consultant. For one thing, eating animal protein washes much more calcium out of the body in the urine than eating soy protein. One study found that women eating meat lost 50 milligrams more calcium per day than when they ate the same amount of protein in soy milk. "A 50-milligram daily difference in calcium loss over twenty years could have a profound detrimental effect on bone mass," says Dr. Messina. Further, animal studies find that soy chemicals have a direct benefit on bone health.

What About Food? To get the antiaging benefits of soybeans, you must eat the beans' protein, as found in soy milk, soy flour, the whole beans, tofu, miso, tempeh and

JAPAN'S ANTIAGING SOUP

Japanese who eat a bowl of miso soup a day cut their risk of fatal stomach cancer by one-third, research has shown. The probable reason: Miso, a fermented soybean product, is an antioxidant, according to experiments at Japan's Okayama University Medical School. In experiments, miso neutralized free radicals and helped protect fats in the body from becoming rancid and able to foment artery clogging. Miso's antioxidant power comes both from common soybean chemicals and from unique substances created by fermentation.

---

textured soy protein. Soy sauce and soybean oil contain very little antiaging compounds. Traces of genistein have been found in other beans, but soybeans have by far the highest concentrations. Incidentally, not all soybeans are white. Recently, genistein was detected in black beans that turned out to be black soybeans.

How Much? Americans eat so little soybean foods that adding any to your diet will undoubtedly help deter aging diseases. The average Asian eats about 50 to 75 milligrams of genistein a day—the amount in about one serving of four ounces of firm or soft tofu. Dr. Messina advises drinking a cup of soy milk or eating three or four ounces of tofu every day.

University of Texas tests reveal that the soybean chemicals genistein and daidzein stay in your body for twenty-four to thirty-six hours. Thus, to keep cells constantly supplied, you need to eat soybean foods every day.

ANTIAGING STRATEGY: HOW TO FEED YOUR CELLS MORE ANTIAGING SOY

- ▲ In baking recipes, use one-third cup of soy flour and two-thirds cup of wheat flour to make one cup of flour.
- ▲ Put defatted soy milk on your cereal, advises cancer researcher John Weisburger, who does just that.
- ▲ Use soy milk instead of cow's milk in recipes for cookies, cakes and puddings.
- ▲ Use soy protein powders to make beverages. One of Dr. Barnes's favorites: one-third cup frozen pina colada mix, one-half cup water and eight ounces of soy protein powder. Stir until powder is dissolved.
- ▲ Use roasted soy nuts as a snack. They are readily available in most grocery stores.
- ▲ Make fruit shakes with tofu or soy milk instead of cow's milk.
- ▲ Add chunks of tofu or tempeh (fermented soybean cake) or both to stir-fried vegetables.
- ▲ Eat imitation meat products—"hot dogs" and "hamburgers" made primarily with soy—for example, frozen Boca burgers and Yves Veggie Wieners; both taste and look remarkably like the real thing.
- ▲ Cook green soybeans as a vegetable.
- ▲ Use dried soybeans as you would other dried beans, such as navy beans. Put them in casseroles, stews and soups.
- ▲ Substitute textured vegetable protein to replace part or all of the ground beef, pork or veal in meat loaf, casseroles, tacos, spaghetti sauce, sloppy joes and chili. TVP or TSP (textured soy

protein), as it's called, comes in granular or chunk form, which when rehydrated resembles ground beef or stew meat.

WHERE TO GET ANTIAGING AGENTS IN SOY FOODS

	MILLIGRAMS OF ISOFLAVONES (GENISTEIN AND DAIDZEIN)
Soy milk: 1 cup	40
Tofu: $1/2$ cup	40
Tempeh: $1/2$ cup	40
Miso: $1/2$ cup	40
Textured vegetable protein, cooked: $1/2$ cup	35
Soy flour: $1/2$ cup	50
Soybeans, cooked: $1/2$ cup	35
Soy nuts: 1 ounce	40

Source: Mark Messina, Ph.D., Virginia Messina, R.D., Kenneth D. R. Setchell, Ph.D., The Simple Soybean and Your Health, *Avery Press, 1994*

The Ancient Longevity Drink

▲　▲　▲

(Why You Need to Drink Tea to Stop Aging)

Drink tea to partake of one of the secrets of the ages. Tea has been known as an extraordinary antiaging drink for four thousand years in Asian cultures. Science now says it's so.

If you literally want to drink from the fountain of youth, drink tea. Tea is an extraordinary drink—mainly because it is made from the leaves of *Camellia sinesis,* a warm-weather evergreen plant, blessed with mixtures of unique antioxidants that are infused into hot water when you make tea. Black tea, green tea, oolong tea, the "real thing"—not herbal teas—can all boost your chances of reaching old age in good shape, according to new research. Drinking antioxidant-packed tea promises to delay aging, prolong life and scare off many chronic diseases, including cancer and heart disease. Although Asian-type green tea contains more of particular types of antioxidants, black tea, popular in Western countries, seems equally effective at defusing free radical attacks on cells, thwarting aging.

Anything that fights off free radicals not only puts you on the aging slow track, but ups your chances of living longer. Indeed, tea appears to be a longevity agent. Two recent studies, one in Norway and one in the Netherlands, both identified tea drinking as insurance against disease and premature death. The Norwegian government study of twenty thousand persons found lower death rates among those who drank at least one cup of tea a day. Similarly, another large-scale government dietary analysis of elderly Dutch men found that those drinking a couple of cups of black tea daily were less apt to die of any cause, but particularly of heart disease. Researchers credited antioxidants, called flavonoids, in the diet, citing tea as the main source.

Prominent cancer researcher Dr. John Weisburger of the American Health Foundation drinks about five cups of tea a day. He says it delivers as much antioxidant punch as two fruits or vegetables.

TEA SECRETS

Tea is a chemical soup of numerous antioxidant polyphenols, such as catechins and quercetin, also concentrated in grapes, berries, onions and red wine. Italian researchers have proved that drinking tea peps up antioxidant activity in your blood by about 50 percent. In a new study, Mauro Serafini at the National Institute of Nutrition in Rome had subjects drink slightly more than a cup of strong tea brewed for two minutes with three teaspoons of either black or green tea leaves. Tests revealed that antioxidant activity in the tea drinkers' blood soared by 41 to 48 percent within thirty minutes after they drank green tea and fifty minutes after they drank black tea. After eighty minutes the antioxidant activity in both green and black tea drinkers returned to normal.

Another powerful way tea works is to rev up the liver's all-important enzyme detoxification system that rids the body of free radicals and other foreign chemicals that damage cells. Black and green tea work equally well, according to tests by John Weisburger, Ph.D., of the American Health Foundation. Tea also neutralizes cell-destroying nitrosamines, derived from cured meats, and heterocyclic amines (HCAs) formed when meat is cooked. That means drinking tea at the same time as eating meat may defuse some of the danger.

HOW TEA CAN FIGHT AGING

Prevents Cardiovascular Deaths: Compelling evidence of tea's powers to ward off fatal heart disease comes from a five-year study of 805 men, aged sixty-five to eighty-four, in the Netherlands. Those who took in the most antioxidant flavonoids, mainly by drinking two cups or more of black tea a day, had only one-half the rate of fatal heart disease as those drinking less tea. Other studies show that tea reduces cholesterol (9 points down in Norwegian men drinking five or more cups a day) and blocks the buildup of plaque in arteries. Tea drinkers also have displayed younger, less damaged arteries at autopsy. Among six thousand Japanese women, those who drank at least five cups of green tea every day had only half the risk of stroke as those who drank less. Further, black tea appears to help dissolve and prevent blood clots and may be as strong as vitamin E at preventing oxidative changes in detrimental LDL cholesterol, leading to artery narrowing and clogging, according to Robert Nicolosi, professor of clinical sciences and tea researcher at the University of Massachusetts.

Stifles Cancer: Animals drinking either green or black tea don't get as much cancer. Nor do humans. A National Cancer Institute study in Shanghai found that men who drank at least one cup of green tea daily slashed their odds of esophageal cancer by 20 percent and women by

50 percent! Nonsmokers and nondrinkers got more protection—up to 60 percent. But don't drink tea boiling hot. It raised the risk of esophageal cancer five times. The hot tea scalds the lining of the esophagus, creating wounds that eventually can become cancerous. Elderly longtime tea drinkers (more than two cups per day) also had an astonishing 63 percent lower risk of pancreatic cancer compared with those who drank less than a cup of tea a day, according to research at the University of Southern California School of Medicine.

Tea even seems to help stop the spread of cancer. Rutgers researchers showed that tea chemicals impeded the ability of leukemia and liver tumor cells to make DNA, necessary to reproduce themselves. Thus, the cancer cells could not proliferate and spread the tumor. Tea works at least five different ways to block both formation and growth of malignant tumors, Rutgers investigators said.

Keeps Gums Healthy: Compounds in both green and black tea combat specific bacterial activity that causes gum tissue destruction or periodontal disease and loss of teeth, according to researchers at Tokyo Dental College. Tea was more powerful at stopping this process than even the common antibiotic tetracycline. Black, oolong and green tea also help prevent cavities, primarily by attacking *Streptococcus mutans,* the main bacteria that cause tooth decay.

> **Drink tea with meals. It helps neutralize cancer causing compounds you take in with food, advises cancer researcher Hans Stich, at the University of British Columbia. "Drinking green tea with meals in Japan and China is thought to be a major reason for low cancer rates in these countries," he says.**

WHEN RED WINE IS NOT YOUR CUP OF TEA

Surprising fact: Drinking tea may give you nearly the identical antioxidant benefits that red wine does. Some tea is even richer in catechins, chemicals regarded as one of red wine's most potent antioxidant weapons. For example, a glass of red wine has 300 milligrams of catechins; a cup of green tea has 375 milligrams of catechins and a cup of black tea contains 210 milligrams, according to tests by Dr. Andrew Waterhouse at the University of California at Davis. So drinking tea should be just as anti-aging as drinking red wine, and safer for many because you don't get the alcohol.

Purple grape juice is another nonalcoholic substitute for red wine. But you must drink three times as much grape juice to get the same antioxidant and anticlogging effect as from red wine.

What Type? Until recently, most research hailed green tea, the type popular in Asia, as stronger in antioxidants than common black tea drunk by most Westerners. True, green tea does contain more of one type antioxidant, called catechins, than black tea. However, new research shows that black tea contains other antioxidants that provide antioxidant activity equal to that of green tea. Thus, black and green teas, as well as oolong tea—the three varieties of real tea—all are effective at defusing free radical attacks on cells, thwarting aging. Black tea is simply green tea leaves that have been dried and heated, changing the color and taste. Oolong tea is partially dried and heated. Instant tea also contains the active ingredients, and iced tea is just as potentially antiaging as hot or warm tea. Tea bags have as much antioxidant power as loose tea, assuming you leave them in the hot water for the same length of time.

How Long to Brew? To extract its maximum antioxidant activity, you should let tea steep in hot water for three minutes, research shows, using one tea bag or one teaspoon of loose tea per cup. Incidentally, nearly all tea's caffeine is released in the first minute of brewing.

The Stuff
That Robs You
of Your Youth

▲   ▲   ▲   ▲   ▲   ▲   ▲

In the elegant dance of life and death between free radicals and antioxidants, it's as important that you don't take in unnecessary cell-damaging free radicals as it is that you take in plenty of antioxidants. Some of the foods and beverages you consume pose dangers to your quest for youth. Here's what you need to know about some of the foods and beverages that can both bestow and rob you of your youth.

Beware the Fat
That Makes You Old

▲ ▲ ▲

(Why You Need to Avoid Certain Fats to Stop Aging)

One of the best ways in the world to stop aging fast is to stop eating fat—not just any kind of fat, but the *wrong kind of fat*!

To be sure, eating fat can make you fat and ruin your arteries. But fat's other crime against humanity is less well known: It makes you old.

Absolutely true. If you want to age fast, eat the type of fat that turns into a free radical factory in your body, making your cells dysfunctional, cancerous, wantonly destructive and suicidal. Eating the wrong fat sets off fierce chain reactions in which free radicals rip through your cells, mutilating and draining them of life. The fats you let into your body are key to how fast you age and the diseases that may overtake you.

Imprint this indelibly into your brain: You can speed up aging or you can slow it down by the type of fat you eat. Here's why:

Oxygen loves fat. Oxygen dissolves eight times faster in fat than in water. And oxygen is more attracted to some fats than others. Fat becomes oxidized when it is exposed to oxygen. If you set a glass of vegetable oil, such as corn oil, in open air, the oil quickly becomes infused with oxygen. "It's incredible how fast this happens—within two or three seconds," says free radical researcher Harry Demopoulos, M.D., formerly a professor at New York University and now president of Antioxidant Pharmaceuticals Corporation in Elmsford, New York.

As the fat takes on oxygen, it becomes progressively rancid or "peroxidized" and ever more dangerous. It is now packed with "lipid hydroperoxide" molecules—some of the ugliest free radicals on the face of the earth. You don't want to take these into your body by eating rancid fat. They are a time bomb, guaranteed to go off inside your cells. Once ingested, the lipid hydroperoxide molecule, encouraged by body warmth, various enzymes and iron and copper, breaks apart, releasing two chemical monsters, including the dreaded hydroxyl radical, that go on rampages of cell destruction. Their trademark: chain reactions that ignite one cell after another, like a burning fuse, turning them into malfunctioning junk, sometimes destroying dozens of cells at a time before being extinguished. This is the stuff aging and disease are made of.

Imagine this kind of free radical havoc in the fragile fatty membranes of your brain cells day after day.

THE FAT FACTS

- ▲ Fat's major crime against humanity is not heart disease or obesity, but overall accelerated aging.
- ▲ Some fats steal your youth faster than others.
- ▲ The worst fats are polyunsaturated fats and cholesterol.
- ▲ The longevity fats are monounsaturated fats, such as olive oil.

The Good, the Bad and the Ugly

A foolproof way to forestall aging: Stop putting rancid fats in your mouth. Unfortunately, rancid fat is an unseen staple in processed foods. Numerous prepackaged foods on supermarket shelves have fat that tends to turn rancid—crackers, cookies, cookie mixes, cakes, cake mixes, chips, pastries, donuts, muffins, frostings, cereals, sauce mixes, dinner mixes, peanut butter, vegetable cooking oils, salad dressings, mayonnaise, pizza and pie crusts, puddings and powdered eggs.

Even fat in frozen foods, such as fried chicken, can oxidize. Cholesterol in meat, eggs and other animal foods also rapidly becomes oxidized. Moreover, during the process of digestion, polyunsaturated fat is further oxidized inside your body as it passes through the intestinal tract.

Not all fats steal your youth equally. Primarily, whether a fat makes you old before your time depends on its chemical affinity for oxygen, how quickly it becomes oxidized. Slowest to oxidize, thus kindest to your cells, are monounsaturated fats, such as olive oil. Cholesterol is bad because it oxidizes readily. The truly ugly fats are the polyunsaturated fats, such as corn oil, that sop up oxygen like crazy, become quickly rancid or oxidized and spew off free radicals.

The result—a flood of alarming consequences, such as damaged DNA in cells and heightened inflammatory responses. Studies show polyunsaturated fats foster auto-immune diseases, encourage cancer, help destroy your arteries and have an adverse effect on your immune functioning. In other words, they create all the hallmarks of premature aging.

Indeed, the more your entire body is filled with rapidly oxidizing and already peroxidized polyunsaturated fats, the more rancid—and more aged—you tend to become. Nature obviously never imagined the mass processing and consumption of such oils that now flood our cells. Yet the rules are firm: You get no more preferential treatment than does a piece of meat lying in the air and sun. Your fat, too, becomes oxidized and you, too, begin to spoil.

As far back as 1954, pioneering free radical researcher Dr. Denham Harman warned that such fats could produce aging and disease, not retard it.

What's the most dangerous fat you can eat?

"Corn oil and safflower oil," says Dr. Harman. The safest? "Olive oil."

A good reason to choose fat-free crackers, cookies, pastries, baked goods—in fact, fat-free everything in processed foods—is to avoid potentially rancid polyunsaturated fats.

WHERE YOU FIND FATS THAT STEAL YOUR YOUTH

To stay young you must restrict omega-6 polyunsaturated fats, such as margarine, shortenings and salad oils made predominantly from corn oil and regular safflower and sunflower seed oil.

Here are the most common edible oils ranked from worst to best by percentages of omega-6 polyunsaturated fatty acids: safflower, regular (77 percent); sunflower, regular (69 percent); corn oil (61 percent); soybean oil (54 percent); walnut oil (51 percent); sesame seed oil (41 percent); peanut oil (33 percent); canola oil (22 percent); flaxseed oil (16 percent); olive oil, extra virgin (8 percent); macadamia nut oil (3 percent). Note: Some safflower and sunflower seed oils have been altered to make them highly monounsaturated instead of polyunsaturated. Check the label.

SUPER PRO-AGING TERRORISTS

As dangerous as omega-6 fats are, they become even worse when they are converted from liquid to solid or semisolid—hydrogenated or partially hydrogenated—as in making margarine and shortening. During the hardening, they take on an additional negative trait, a kinky new form, unknown in nature, changing them into trans fatty acids, abhorrent to your body. Basically, your body is then forced to create additional floods of free radicals in efforts to metabolize or digest these abnormal fats.

The way trans fats mangle your cell membranes is not a pretty picture. Such fatty molecules packed tightly into the membranes of your cells make them rigid, inflexible and essentially dysfunctional. Such warped cells can no longer circulate easily in surveillance teams to rally immune defenses to fight off infections or destroy tumor cells. They are so stiff they can't do the mundane job of encircling bacteria, viruses and cancer cells to destroy them. "It's sort of like lock-jaw. They can't open their mouths to swallow them up," says Dr. Demopoulos. Nor can they slip easily through narrowed arteries to keep blood flowing to the heart and brain.

Some specific documented crimes of trans fatty acids: They disturb heart rhythms, help clog arteries by encouraging "sticky" blood; lower good HDL cholesterol; increase bad LDL and lipoprotein Lp(a), another hazardous blood factor; depress immune functioning; produce abnormal sperm and lower testosterone in animals; promote cancer, notably breast and prostate cancer. Indeed, Harvard's Dr. Walter Willett suspects these fats, rather than saturated animal fats, are a prime cause of our skyrocketing rates of heart disease. He notes that Americans' intake of trans fatty acids from hydrogenated vegetable fats zoomed from zero in 1900 to 5.5 percent of our total fat consumption in the 1960s. Was it mere coincidence that this unprecedented trans fatty acid binge closely paralleled our soaring rates of coronary heart disease? Dr. Willett thinks not.

Generally, studies show that processed high-fat foods, such as cakes, cookies, corn chips, donuts and potato chips, have the highest levels of trans fatty acids.

MARGARINE: A SPECIAL DOOMSDAY THREAT

It's almost incredible that Americans' number-one source of fat by far is margarine. Perhaps that helps explain why we are number seventeen among nations in life expectancy. Margarine in the United States is also the prime carrier of trans fatty acids that make cells so grotesque they cannot function normally.

A Harvard study by Dr. Willett found that women who ate four or more teaspoons of margarine a day had a 66 percent higher risk of heart disease than women who ate less than one teaspoon a month. A Greek study found that cooking with margarine increased the risk of heart disease by nearly 90 percent. Dr. Willett's studies also suggest that women who eat high levels of trans fatty acids are more vulnerable to breast cancer and men are more prone to prostate cancer. And, of course, anything that burdens your body with more free radicals is responsible for a much longer list of sins, including premature aging.

Eating trans fatty acids, particularly margarine, kills from thirty thousand to one hundred fifty thousand Americans every year from heart disease. —Walter Willett, M.D., Harvard School of Public Health

---

FATS THAT MAKE YOU OLD

▲ Highly polyunsaturated fats such as corn, safflower, sunflower seed, peanut oils.
▲ Margarine and shortening (trans fatty acids).
▲ Cholesterol.
▲ Animal fats in meat, poultry, dairy products.

FATS THAT KEEP YOU YOUNG

▲ Olive oil.
▲ Canola oil.
▲ Macadamia nut oil.
▲ Fish oil.
▲ Flaxseed oil.

Whenever you see these words on a food label ingredients—"hydrogenated" or "partially hydrogenated" vegetable oil, especially as the first ingredient, it's cause for alarm. It's another word for trans fatty acids. Hardened stick margarine, the most highly hydrogenated, is worst; softer tub and liquid margarine are lower in trans fatty acids, but are still a concentrated source of omega-6 polyunsaturated danger. However, it's always much safer to consume vegetable oils of all types in their natural state—not solidified.

CHOLESTEROL: AGENT OF PREMATURE AGING

High-cholesterol foods also steal your youth. Eating foods high in cholesterol may not sound so scary when all they threaten to do is maybe raise your blood cholesterol—and usually not much. But what if you knew that cholesterol-packed eggs, meat and cheese also promote aging? A large epidemiological study by Richard Shekelle, Ph.D., professor of epidemiology at the University of Texas Health Science Center in Houston, found that high-cholesterol eaters (700 milligrams or more a day) cut an average three years off their life spans. He also discovered that high-cholesterol eaters were more apt to develop lung cancer.

It's probably due to the free radical thugs. Cholesterol in foods reacts readily with oxygen to form cholesterol oxidized products or COP, also called "rusty cholesterol." These are extremely potent free radicals. They can damage the DNA of cells irreparably. In one experiment, scientists bathed the aorta of rabbits in these COPs and then peered through an electromicroscope to observe the damage. The free radical reactions from the COP had eaten holes in the outer lining of the aorta, according to Dr. Demopoulos. Such tiny holes in arteries are an invitation for platelets and debris to pile up, starting the formation of plaque, leading to clogged arteries.

What's worse, some high-cholesterol foods, mainly meat, are also rich in iron—a fearsome combination. Iron cuddles up to cholesterol and acts as a catalyst for free radical reactions. So cholesterol mated with iron in the same food and dropped into the intestinal tract can create loads of rusty cholesterol molecules to attack your cells.

THE BEST ANTIOXIDANT FAT

Use olive oil (and other monounsaturated fats) to preserve youth and stave off disease and death. Mono fats are slow to oxidize or turn rancid, and also actively help curb free radical reactions. Not surprisingly, olive oil eaters tend to have less cancer and heart disease. Harvard researchers found that women in Greece who ate olive oil more than once a day had 25 percent lower breast cancer rates than women eating olive oil less frequently. Eating at least two teaspoons of olive oil daily cut the risk of breast cancer by 30 to 35 percent in Spanish women.

In Mediterranean countries high olive oil consumption is tied to much lower rates of heart disease. Exciting experiments by Peter Reaven and colleagues at the University of California, as well as in Israel, reveal one reason: Monounsaturated fats actually deter oxidation of bad-type LDL cholesterol; thus, the cholesterol can't penetrate artery walls, creating gunk that rots arteries and triggers heart attacks and strokes. Such mono fats also lower detrimental LDL cholesterol and boost the efficiency of good type HDL cholesterol in ridding the body of LDL cholesterol. Further, antioxidant vitamin E works better to fight free radicals in your cells if monounsaturated type fat is also present. So for maximum antiaging vitamin E benefits, it's best to eat olive oil and other mono fats.

Famous cholesterol researcher Ancel Keys summed up the case for monounsaturated fats and olive oil about a decade ago. He documented that Mediterranean peoples who use olive oil as their prime source of fat have the lowest mortality rates; they are least likely to die of anything!

Antiaging foods rich in monounsaturated fat include olive oil, macadamia nut oil, flaxseed oil, olives, avocados, almonds and hazelnuts.

FISH OIL—A MIGHTY YOUTH POTION

To save your cells, especially from domination by the harmful omega-6 fats, be sure to eat so-called omega-3 fatty acids. You get them in fatty fish, such as salmon, mackerel

and sardines, as well as in some plant foods—flaxseed, walnuts and soybeans. These unique omega-3 fats overthrow
the little dictators—the omega-6 fats—that otherwise rule
the activity of your cells, causing continual injury. You want
as much omega-3s in your cells as omega-6s, according to
experts. Unfortunately, most Americans have ten to twenty
times more omega-6s than omega-3s in their cells from
being gluttons for margarine and other such fats.

Such an imbalance fosters many woes of aging, such
as arthritis, lung damage, strokes, heart irregularities, diabetes and various types of cancer. For example, animal
studies at Dartmouth Medical School by Dr. Bill D. Roe-
buck show that feeding animals omega-3 fat deters pancreatic cancer, but omega-6 oils, in amounts commonly
found in our diet, enhance pancreatic cancer.

New research at New York Cornell Medical Center also
finds that in animals omega-3 fat actually revs up
enzymes, including glutathione S transferase, to fight off
free radicals and generally detoxify the body. It works
much the same way as anticancer chemicals in broccoli.

It's instructive to note that fish eaters throughout the
world tend to have less cancer and heart disease and to
live longer than non–fish eaters. Fish's unique fat, experts
believe, is a prime reason. (For more on the antiaging
properties of fish, see page 182.)

How Animal Fat Steals Your Youth

Another demon fat is saturated animal fat, as in meat,
poultry, whole milk, cheese and butter. This is the type of
fat that ruins your arteries in numerous ways. Saturated fat
is the main culprit in boosting your bad-type LDL blood
cholesterol. It also suppresses clot-dissolving activity and
causes blood to become more sticky and apt to form clots,

STOP AGING NOW! —

THE TWO FACES OF SOYBEANS

Most of the harmful fat in processed foods comes from partially hydrogenated soybean oil. However, liquid soybean oil does have some redeeming value: It contains moderate amounts of beneficial omega-3 fatty acids. Also, the body tends to chemically change soybean oil into beneficial omega-3 type fat. However, lots of harmful omega-6s are still left over.

In contrast to soybean oil, soy protein foods, such as plain soybeans, tofu and soy milk contain substances, such as genistein, known as strong antioxidants and cancer fighters.

Avoid hydrogenated soybean oils, go easy on plain soybean oil, and embrace soy protein foods (see page 189).

precipitating heart attacks and strokes. Saturated animal fat also influences hormones, promoting breast cancer and prostate cancer. Women who eat lots of animal fat generally have higher levels of circulating estradiol, a cancer promoter. Research consistently shows that people who eat more fat, namely animal fat, have much more colon cancer. In one Harvard study, men who ate the least saturated fat (7 percent of calories in animal fat) had half the rate of precancerous polyps compared with men who ate twice that much (14 percent of calories in saturated fat.) These polyps can progress to become full-blown tumors.

Moreover, animal fat stimulates production of inflammatory agents in the body, called prostaglandins and leukotrienes. These can cause widespread destruction of joints, promoting rheumatoid arthritis; such inflammation is also incriminated in artery clogging, migraine headaches and psoriasis.

The type of fat you eat can also rev up or depress your entire detoxification system, including the way you handle free radicals. This affects your health on a global scale, influencing susceptibility not only to cancer, but to heart disease, high blood pressure, autoimmune and inflammatory diseases, liver disease and, of course, aging in general.

Based on animal studies done at Strang Cancer Prevention Center in New York, saturated fat, especially butter, is most likely to suppress this all-important detoxification system by switching certain genes on or off. In contrast, fish oil (omega-3) powerfully stimulates enzyme detoxification machinery, according to Andrew J. Dannenberg, M.D., director of the center. Liquid soybean oil also revved up detoxification enzymes to a lesser degree, but hydrogenated or hardened soybean oil suppressed it. This shows how the face of soybean oil can change from benevolent to vicious when its chemistry is changed to form trans fatty acids.

How to Keep Fats from Spoiling Your Youth

- ▲ Eat as little peroxidized or rancid fat as possible.
- ▲ Check the label of processed foods; if it lists polyunsaturated fats such as safflower oil, sunflower seed oil, corn oil, soybean oil or peanut oil, it has assuredly been oxidized to a degree.
- ▲ Particularly shun foods that contain hydrogenated or partially hydrogenated vegetable oils (trans fatty acids).

▲ Opt for fat-free crackers, cookies, baked goods and cereals. You can be sure these do not have rancid fats.

▲ Primarily use extra virgin olive oil and canola oil for cooking and making salad dressings. Macadamia nut and walnut oil are also good.

▲ Restrict animal foods high in saturated fat and cholesterol, such as pork, beef, lamb, veal, poultry skin, butter, whole milk, cheese and full-fat yogurt.

▲ Eat fish; it contains both omega-3 fats as well as antioxidants that tend to block oxidation of fat.

▲ Eat fruits and vegetables high in glutathione and/or take glutathione and glutamine supplements to help defuse fat's free radical activity. Glutathione is a Rambo-like antioxidant that helps neutralize rancid fats in the intestinal tract, curbing their free radical activity. (See page 124.)

Curing Meat of Its Youth-Stealing Powers

▲　▲　▲

(How You Can Eat Meat and Still Stop Aging)

Eating meat sabotages your cells—promoting aging along with heart damage and cancer. But some simple measures, including the way you cook meat, can help curb the damage.

It's not just fat in meat and poultry that make them an aging threat. Meat has other hidden hazards that can steal your youth and vigor and hasten the onset of major diseases associated with aging, namely cancer and heart disease. But the good news is, if you don't want to give up meat entirely, you can dramatically diminish meat-generated attacks on cells, partially defusing the pro-aging damage.

When you cook meat, poultry and even fish to a much lesser extent, substances called HCAs (heterocyclic amines) are created. These HCAs are born of reactions with animal proteins during the browning process. But they are not on the surface of the meat. Thus, you cannot scrape off the char of a burger or barbecued chicken and be rid of them. HCAs arise from heat-induced reactions within the muscle and are actually embedded in cooked meat. However, the temperature at which you cook meat makes a big difference. Cooking such meats at high temperatures as in frying, grilling, broiling and barbecuing produces loads of the nasty chemicals. Oven roasting and baking produce fewer HCAs, and stewing, boiling, poaching and microwaving generate virtually no HCAs.

Fortunately, the danger is not nearly as great in cooked fish. One study found that frying chicken and beef produced five to eight times more HCAs than frying fish. The most HCAs are found in fried bacon, and, not surprisingly, regularly eating fried bacon raises your risk of heart disease and cancer.

Free Radical Monsters on the Loose

Make no mistake about it, HCAs are powerful mutagens that can stimulate free radicals and extensively damage cells' genetic material (DNA). In animals, HCAs cause colon, breast, pancreatic, liver and bladder cancer. Some are "extraordinarily efficient and rapid" at inducing liver cancer in monkeys, our closest relatives, says researcher Dr. John Weisburger of the American Health Foundation. People who eat broiled and fried meats are more apt to develop colon cancer. HCAs may be partly responsible for increased colon and breast cancer in women who eat meat, along with the typical American high-fat diet.

When fat was discounted, one study found that women who ate meat—beef, veal, lamb, pork—every day were still about twice as likely to develop breast cancer as women eating mostly fish and poultry, according to a study at New York University Medical Center. Women who ate five ounces of lamb, pork or beef a day had twice the odds of colon cancer as women eating it less than once a month, according to a Harvard study. Primary targets of HCAs as cancer threats are the colon, breast and pancreas.

HCAs can also attack the heart. After observing severe

heart damage in monkeys with liver cancer due to HCAs, Cindy D. Davis and colleagues at the National Cancer Institute did some experiments. They found that certain HCAs destroyed the mitochondria in heart muscle cells, triggering cell death. The mitochondria are energy factories, essential to cell survival. Such destruction, Davis speculates, might be involved in cardiomyopathy, a characteristic disease of aging in which heart tissue becomes inflamed and deteriorates, often eventually resulting in heart failure.

Nothing is more hazardous to your youth than attacks on the mitochondria. Such destruction of the cell's mitochondria is thought to be the primary underlying cause of overall premature aging.

ANTIAGING SECRETS OF THE EXPERTS

William Castelli, M.D.:
Heart Disease Explorer

Dr. Castelli is director of the famed Framingham (Massachusetts) Heart Study.

"I'm the first member of my family to make it past age forty-five without coronary heart disease."

Here's what he takes every day:

- ▲ Vitamin C—500 milligrams.
- ▲ Vitamin E—400 IU.
- ▲ Folic acid–1 milligram (1,000 micrograms).
- ▲ Multivitamin-mineral supplement—1 tablet.

NEW CANCER THREATS IN MEAT

Another big danger in meat, unrelated to fat, is the potential formation of nitrosamines, chemicals that can cause virtually every type of cancer. Nitrosamines can form inside the stomach after eating sodium nitrite in cured meats, such as ham, hot dogs, bologna, salami and other cold cuts, and bacon. Further, nitrosamines are already often preformed in meats, such as bacon, needing no further bodily chemical reactions to make them potentially hazardous.

Some recent disturbing evidence links cured meats to various cancers.

Brain Cancer: Researchers at the University of North Carolina at Chapel Hill recently discovered that youngsters who ate hot dogs once a week or more had twice the risk of brain tumor compared with non–hot dog eating kids. Moreover, youngsters eating the most other cured meats, such as ham, bacon and sausage, had an 80 percent higher risk of brain cancer. Of utmost interest: Kids taking vitamins were less vulnerable to the brain cancer, suggesting that the antioxidant vitamins countered free radicals and carcinogens in the cured meats.

Leukemia: Hot dogs are tied to childhood leukemia, according to research at the University of Southern California School of Medicine in Los Angeles. Youngsters eating more than twelve hot dogs a month had nearly ten times the risk of leukemia as kids who ate none. The most likely culprit is nitrite and nitrate used to cure the meats, said researchers.

RECIPE FOR AN ANTIAGING HAMBURGER

One amazing way to slash HCA hazards in burgers is to mix in soy protein before cooking. Tests by researcher Dr. John Weisburger show that an incredibly small amount of soy protein—as little as 10 percent by weight of a mixture of ground meat—blocks the formation of cell-damaging, cancer-causing HCAs when you cook the hamburger. The soy also replaces some of the hazardous fat. If the standard hamburger around the world were made with even a little soy, cancer rates worldwide would drop, suggests Dr. Weisburger.

Here's his recipe for an antiaging hamburger: Mix one-half cup of textured vegetable protein granules (a form of soy protein available in health food stores and some supermarkets) and two tablespoons of cold water with a pound of lean ground beef. Knead meat until all the ingredients are combined. Form into patties and cook. The soy eliminates about 95 percent of the HCAs. Thus, the soy-hamburger has only 5 percent of the hazardous HCAs found in an ordinary hamburger! There is no noticeable difference in taste or texture.

Colon Cancer: Eating processed meats, namely sausage, hiked colon cancer risk, according to a Dutch study of about thirty-seven hundred men and women. The researchers primarily blamed sausage's curing agents.

The Iron Connection? Meat is also high in iron, which can foster production of cell-damaging free radicals in your body. Iron has been incriminated specifically in colon and breast cancer and heart disease.

Extra danger: Fat and cholesterol in meat also trigger free radicals that promote many aging diseases, including cancer, clogged arteries and inflammatory problems, including arthritis.

ANTIAGING STRATEGY: DEFUSING MEAT'S PRO-AGING TIME BOMB

Counter with Antioxidants: When you eat meat of any kind, be sure to eat plenty of high antioxidant foods, such as fruits, vegetables, grains and tea at the same meal or around the same time. And take vitamins as insurance to keep blood levels of antioxidants high. Studies show antioxidant vitamins C, E and A, carotene, selenium, glutathione and tea compounds can help neutralize the formation of HCAs along with other cell-destroying free radicals. Vitamin C in fruits and vegetables and vitamin E also block formation of nitrosamines. So do garlic, green peppers, pineapple, carrots, strawberries and tomatoes, according to tests at Cornell University. The nitrosamine-blocking antioxidants in fruits and vegetables are many, including quercetin, p-coumaric and chlorogenic acids as well as vitamin C, researchers have found.

Eat Garlic: New studies have found that garlic not only can prevent formation of dreaded nitrosamines that can come from eating cured meats, but also can block the intact nitrosamine molecule from becoming biologically activated and thus dangerous to cells.

Cook Meat in Ways to Reduce Danger: Preferably microwave, stew, boil and poach meat and poultry, methods that create very few HCAs. If you do grill, first microwave burgers, chops, steaks and poultry to cook them partially.

Then before putting them on the grill, drain and discard their juices, which are rich in raw materials to produce HCAs. Tests by James S. Felton, at Lawrence Livermore National Laboratory in California, showed that pre-cooking a hamburger in the microwave for two minutes before putting it on the grill reduced the HCAs 90 percent compared with simply slapping a raw burger on the grill. Also, don't use meat drippings to make gravy; such gravy will contain high concentrations of HCAs.

Always microwave bacon. Bacon cooked in the microwave has fewer nitrosamines and HCAs than fried or broiled bacon.

Remove Fat: Trim fat off meat before cooking or eating it. Don't eat poultry skin.

Eat Smaller Portions of Meats: Instead of a customary serving of twelve ounces of steak or roast beef or an eight-ounce hamburger, use smaller portions of three and a half to four ounces.

Restrict Meat Intake: Making meat the centerpiece of every meal is a good way to grow old fast. Substitute main dishes of vegetables, grains, pastas and legumes. Mix smaller amounts of meat into casseroles and into stir-fries as Asian cooks do. If you are a once- or twice-a-day meat eater, at least try to cut down to having meat only three or four times a week. As President Thomas Jefferson once said, meat should be a side dish to the main course of potatoes, rice, vegetables and legumes.

Drinking Yourself Young or Old

▲ ▲ ▲

(What You Need to Know
About Alcohol to Stop Aging)

Drinking a little alcohol, particularly red wine, can be a prescription for youth—if you are an adult and have no problems or conditions that would rule out alcohol. Drinking a lot is a fast way to make yourself old, damaged and dead.

The truth is, you can drink yourself young and you can drink yourself old. And the margin of difference is very slim. Dozens of studies show that "moderate" drinkers of alcohol, one or two drinks a day on average, live slightly longer than teetotalers, but "heavy" drinkers—more than three daily drinks—die faster than anybody. It's tough to ignore the evidence. For example, a thirteen-year-long study of twelve thousand male British physicians, ages fifty to ninety, reported in 1994 by the Imperial Cancer Research Fund at Oxford University, found that moderate drinkers lived about two years longer than nondrinkers. They also found that the chances of death accelerated the more alcohol the doctors drank in excess of three drinks a day. Imbibers of more than six drinks a day were most apt to have cirrhosis, liver cancer, mouth and throat cancer, bronchitis and pneumonia.

Does that mean you should drink specifically to post-

THE STUFF THAT ROBS YOU OF YOUR YOUTH —

THE ANTIAGING FACTS ABOUT ALCOHOL

▲ Alcohol in moderation may prolong life primarily by fighting heart disease after middle age.

▲ Wine is most apt to lessen heart attacks, beer next and hard liquor least, according to a recent study at Kaiser Permanente in California.

▲ Best antiaging bet, if you drink, is to drink wine with meals. Knocking down drinks at a bar or party without significant amounts of food is a good way to kill your youth and yourself fast.

pone aging? Definitely not. But if you already drink moderately, neither need you stop for fear it will send you prematurely to your grave. As leading cardiologist Thomas Pearson, of Mary Imogen Bassett Research Institute in Cooperstown, New York, told his colleagues: "Generalized messages to abstain from alcohol are probably no more responsible than generalized recommendations to drink it." His point: Whether to drink must be an individual decision based on an adult's attitude toward and experience with alcohol use.

The difference between drinking small and large amounts (of alcohol) may be the difference between preventing and causing premature deaths. —Dr. Charles Hennekens, professor, Harvard Medical School

How Moderate Drinking May Postpone Aging

Reduces Heart Attacks: Typically, people who drink no more than two drinks a day have a 30 percent lower risk of heart disease than nondrinkers. In the recent British physician study, heart attacks and strokes sank 40 percent among moderate drinkers compared with nondrinkers or heavy drinkers. Probable reasons: Alcoholic beverages discourage the formation of blood clots, boost good-type HDL cholesterol and help prevent dreaded oxidation of LDL cholesterol that eventually rots and clogs arteries.

If every American stopped drinking entirely, there would be eighty-one thousand more heart disease deaths a year, predicted Harvard cardiologist Dr. Paul Ridker. He found that daily moderate drinkers have high levels of a natural clot buster called t-PA or tissue-type plasminogen activator. Nondrinkers had the lowest levels of the clot buster.

Wards Off Strokes: Presumably because of its clot-fighting properties, a drink or two a day seems to reduce strokes— by 60 to 70 percent when compared with not drinking at all, according to a recent British study.

Preserves Mental Abilities: Strange as it seems, moderate drinking may also help keep your brain alert as you age. Medical geneticist Joe C. Christian at Indiana University tracked nearly four thousand male twins for twenty years to find out if moderate drinking damaged the brain. He gave psychological tests to the brothers when they were ages sixty-six and seventy-six. He found no harm from a little alcohol. In fact, he discovered that the brothers who drank one or two drinks a day scored higher on mental skills tests than those who drank either less than one drink or more than two drinks. Moderate drinking—from one to two drinks daily—seemed to improve memory, problem solving and reasoning ability.

———

How much? For adults age sixty-five and under, men should have no more than two daily drinks and women, no more than one drink. (Men are generally larger than women and can metabolize more alcohol.) After age sixty-five, no more than one daily drink is advisable for everyone. —National Institute on Alcohol Abuse and Alcoholism

———

How Heavy Drinking Can Steal Your Youth and Cut Your Life Short

Triggers Premature Death: The death toll from alcohol is enormous. Heavy drinking is the second leading cause of "premature" death—smoking is number one. Among participants in the famous Framingham Heart Study, those who consumed more than five or six daily drinks died more often of sudden cardiac arrest, although they did not have signs of coronary heart disease. Alcohol also increases the death toll from high blood pressure; strokes; cancers of the stomach, throat and possibly breast and colon; cirrhosis of the liver; accidents and suicides.

Heavy drinking is the second leading cause of all premature deaths—those before you reach your average expected life span—in the United States. Smoking is first.

Promotes Breast Cancer: More than one drink a day can promote breast cancer, many experts now warn. The culprit may be free radical damage. In one study, Dr. Matthew P. Longnecker at the Harvard School of Public Health determined that drinking roughly a couple of drinks a day boosted the risk of breast cancer about 50 percent. He found one drink a day or less relatively safe.

Women, especially those with a family history of breast cancer, should restrict alcohol to an average of one drink a day. If you have breast cancer, binge drinking could help spread the cancer. Alcohol boosts levels of estrogen that promotes cancer.

Induces Cardiovascular Disease: People who drink three or more drinks a day are three to four times more apt to have high blood pressure. In fact, excessive drinking accounts for up to 30 percent of all cases of high blood pressure, studies show. Heavy drinkers (three to four drinks daily) are three to six times more likely to have a stroke than nondrinkers, according to British and Finnish research. Even in young people, binge drinking can trigger strokes.

Further, chronic heavy drinking can cause irregular heartbeats and enlargement of the heart, leading to shortness of breath and fatigue and eventually congestive heart failure, which is often fatal.

Alcohol is astonishing—it's a potent pharmacologic agent that can be part of a healthy diet and can also be essentially fatal if consumed in excess. —Dr. Walter Willett, Harvard School of Public Health

---

Causes Brain Damage: Unquestionably, alcohol can prematurely age your brain, primarily impairing memory.

WHO SHOULD AVOID ALCOHOL ENTIRELY

▲ Women pregnant or trying to conceive.

▲ People who plan to drive or perform other activities requiring unimpaired attention or muscular coordination.

▲ People taking medications that can interact with alcohol.

▲ Recovering alcoholics.

▲ Children and teenagers.

▲ People with medical conditions that would be worsened by alcohol.

—*National Institute on Alcohol Abuse and Alcoholism*

Scans of the brains of young alcoholics reveal brain damage, including shrinkage of the cortex, impaired cerebral structures and decreased metabolic activity. "The brain of a thirty-year-old alcoholic looks like the brain of a fifty-year-old," says researcher Gene-Jack Wang, M.D., Brookhaven National Laboratory in Upton, New York.

Causes Birth Defects: For pregnant women, drinking alcohol can induce miscarriage, fetal alcohol syndrome and birth defects.

Causes Addiction: Of course, the main youth and life-threatening hazard of alcohol is that many individuals become addicted to it and cannot stop drinking, once they start. About fourteen million adult Americans are hooked on alcohol.

It would be entirely irresponsible to advise non-drinkers to drink for their health. —Arthur Klatsky, chief of cardiology at Kaiser Permanente Medical Center in Oakland, California

RED WINE'S SPECIAL ANTIAGING POWERS

Why is red wine more antiaging than other forms of alcohol? Simple. Red wine has lots of antioxidants. You've probably heard of the French Paradox. It claims the French can eat a lot of fat without suffering a smidgen of the heart disease Americans and other Westerners do because the French drink red wine with meals, which counteracts the expected arterial damage from fatty foods. Whether this is true is controversial, but it is certain that antioxidants are plentiful in wine, particularly red wine, and they do enter your bloodstream in large quantities when you drink wine.

White wine has some antioxidants, but red wine has far more because during the fermentation of red wine, but not white wine, the colorful skins and seeds, the source of the antioxidants, are left in the mix, and the antioxidants are released into the finished wine. One of red wine's greatest antioxidant weapons is a specific compound, known as catechins, also present in tea.

These catechins have wide-ranging benefits: They can block oxidative changes that allow LDL cholesterol to infiltrate artery walls, promoting clogging; inhibit platelet aggregation that foments blood clots; relax blood vessels, inhibit tumors, bacteria and viruses; help protect the liver and fight inflammation.

How Red Wine May Fight Aging

Blocks Artery Clogging: Remarkably, the antioxidants in red grapes and red wine, like vitamin E, thwart free radicals' ability to oxidize your bad-type LDL blood cholesterol that sets the stage for artery clogging. In test-tube experiments, Edwin Frankel, Ph.D., and colleagues at the University of California at Davis found that antioxidants in red wine were even stronger than vitamin E at blocking oxidation. White wine (and green grapes) were not as effective because they have lower levels of antioxidants.

> *I eat more red grapes now and have switched from white wine to red wine.* —Dr. Edwin Frankel, University of California at Davis, antioxidant researcher on wine and grapes

Acts as an Anticoagulant: Antioxidants in red wine act somewhat like aspirin to deter blood platelet clumping, a first step to forming clots, leading to heart attacks and strokes. In recent research by John Folts at the University of Wisconsin–Madison Medical School, subjects drank two and a half glasses of a French red wine (Chateauneuf du Pape). Forty-five minutes later, blood tests showed a drop in platelet stickiness of about 40 percent, meaning they were less vulnerable to blood clots.

Dilates Arteries: Chemicals in red wine, red grapes and red grape juice can even directly affect blood vessels, by relaxing and dilating them, according to tests by David F. Fitzpatrick, Ph.D., at the University of South Florida College of Medicine. This activity may fend off high blood pressure and vascular spasms that precipitate heart attacks and strokes. White grapes and white grape juice also had some effects, but not white wine. The muscle-relaxing chemical is definitely in the grape skin, not the pulp, and may be catechins, says Dr. Fitzpatrick.

INFUSIONS OF PROTECTION

No question, the antioxidant catechins in red wine get into your blood, presumably protecting arteries by their presence, according to Andrew Waterhouse, Ph.D., at the University of California at Davis. He had subjects drink two six-ounce glasses of a red California Bordeaux; their blood levels of catechins jumped dramatically, peaking in three hours. The antioxidants started declining after eight hours and nearly disappeared within twenty-four hours. "It lasted almost a day," marveled Dr. Waterhouse. More remarkably, the amount of catechins in the blood, as extrapolated from test-tube studies, would be expected to reduce dangerous oxidation of LDL cholesterol by 80 percent!

Question: Do all red wines contain antioxidant catechins? Yes, says Dr. Waterhouse. Although some red wines have slightly more catechins, any red wine contains quite a lot, including any ordinary American, French, Italian, Australian, Chilean—you name it—red wine. Which have the most? "If a wine is robust, really gets your mouth puckered up when you drink it, you know there's a lot in there," says Dr. Waterhouse.

TWO NOTES OF CRUCIAL ADVICE

▲ Red wine is not a medicine to be tossed down
   alone any old time you think of it. "If you start
   treating red wine like a pill, you could seriously
   hurt yourself," warns Dr. Waterhouse. If you do

drink red wine, do it the way the French do, with meals. This not only discourages intoxication, but also exploits the wine's potential benefits. The antioxidants in red wine may work primarily by acting as partial antidotes to free radical activity generated by food, notably fatty foods. So having the bad guys and good guys in your body at the same time is what makes the beneficial difference.

▲ More is not better. Drink red wine only in moderation. That means one or two glasses a day. Carrying the wine theory to extremes is dangerous. The French, who drink about ten times more red wine than Americans do, admittedly have low death rates from heart disease. But twice as many Frenchmen die of cirrhosis of the liver, stomach cancer and suicide as their American counterparts. And the death rate for stroke is 50 percent higher for Frenchmen than for American males. Such problems are often alcohol-related.

"Wine" Without the Alcohol

Surprisingly, plain old purple grape juice contains many of the same protective blood-thinning antioxidants as red wine but in lower concentrations, according to new tests by the University of Wisconsin's Dr. John Folts. This means you can get many of the benefits of red wine without the alcohol. You must drink three times as much purple grape juice as red wine to get the same anticoagulant benefits. To counteract the pro-clogging activity of certain fatty foods, it's best to drink the grape juice with meals. White grape juice doesn't work.

The Path to Old Age
Is Paved with Calories

▲ ▲ ▲

(Why Cutting Calories Can Stop Aging)

Even if you are already middle-aged or more, gradually whittling away a few calories every day could slow down your biological clock and delay or save you from the diseases of aging. It's never too late to begin to stave off aging.

Here's a way, although not always agreeable, to slow down aging, avoid disease and add years to your life: Eat fewer calories, but make them high quality, so you are lean but not malnourished. The strategy makes absolute biological sense; it's an almost perfect life extender in animals and it helps explain why certain humans thrive and stay alive much longer than others. Consider the islanders on Japanese Okinawa; they have more citizens over age one hundred than any other population. They eat 17 to 40 percent fewer calories than other Japanese and have 30 to 40 percent less heart disease, stroke, cancer, diabetes and age-related brain disease.

Although Americans are getting fatter, compelling new evidence suggests that eating less is one way to the fountain of youth. According to Roy Walford, director of the Gerontology Research Laboratory at the UCLA Medical School, a low-calorie, high-nutritive diet slows the rate of aging, "rejuvenates" some bodily systems even late in life, stretches life span and cuts susceptibility to disease at least in half.

Does this mean a lifetime of semistarvation? No. Undernutrition, not malnutrition, is the key.

THE ANIMAL CENTENARIANS

Restricting calories is the one absolute surefire, proven way to make animals overshoot their normal life spans. Since the first experiment in 1935, a string of studies shows that mammals, such as mice, rats and dogs, on restricted diets live one-third to one-half longer than expected. It's indisputable that eating 30 to 40 percent less than mammals would otherwise gobble up, along with adequate nutrients, is a virtual guarantee of slower aging. The animals are more frisky, leaner and younger-looking, and less prone to all diseases, including cancer and infections. When cancer is induced in the animals, the tumors often refuse to grow and the ones that do progress at only two-thirds the usual pace.

You can extend longevity by restricting food even after full adulthood and middle age. —Dr. Roy Walford, UCLA School of Medicine

---

Everything we associate with aging is postponed when the brakes are put on calories: puberty is delayed, reproductive life is extended, memory loss and faltering immunity are delayed. The animals are often only half the biological age of animals their same chronological age.

WHY YOU CAN STOP AGING BY RESTRICTING CALORIES

You Produce Fewer Free Radicals: Essentially, calories are the enemies of youth because converting them into energy requires more oxygen that triggers more free radicals that then attack cells, potentially leading to cell damage, disease and accelerated aging. It is a vicious circle; the more you eat, the more oxygen you must process and the more cell damage you can expect. Restricting calories cuts down on destructive free radical production. When the bodies of calorie-restricted animals are measured at death, they show signs of less free radical damage to tissues. They are not as "rusted out" as well-fed animals that die at the same age.

Your Antiaging Defenses Go Up: Underfeeding animals dramatically boosts levels of internally produced antioxidant enzymes, including all-important superoxide dismutase, catalase and glutathione peroxidase—the same vital stuff that bestowed youth and longevity on fruit flies (see page 18). And the enzymes are three to four times more active in neutralizing free radicals, says Ron Hart of the National Center for Toxicological Research in Arkansas. Additionally, calorie-restricted animals dispatch larger enzyme forces to repair genetic (DNA) damage in cells. And they are five times better at flushing carcinogens such as aflatoxin out of their bodies.

Your Immunity Improves: Calorie-restricted animals have one-third stronger immune systems than normal animals, says microbiologist George Roth at the National Institute on Aging. Caloric restriction clearly "delays the drop in immune response that occurs with age, and the potency of white blood cells lasts longer in underfed animals," he says.

Your Blood Sugar and Insulin Levels Drop: Undereating causes a dramatic drop in blood glucose (sugar) and the hormone insulin. That's critical because high circulating blood sugar and insulin are prime biomarkers of aging. If you eat a lot, your body must generate more insulin to convert the food into blood sugar. Insulin is a newly recognized villain in several chronic diseases. It is a coconspirator with fats in the destruction of artery walls, triggering heart disease. It's also a suspected growth promoter of cancer. Too much insulin also can have dire effects on the brain.

BEATING THE BIOLOGICAL CLOCK

Here are the antiaging benefits to monkeys that ate 30 percent fewer calories than normal for forty-two months:

- Lower weight and body fat.
- Lower metabolic rate.
- Lower fasting blood sugar.
- Increased glucose tolerance.
- Lower insulin blood levels.
- Greater insulin sensitivity.
- Lower diastolic and mean blood pressure.
- More lymphocytes (white blood cells) to fight infections.
- Slightly lower cholesterol.

YES, IT WORKS IN HUMANS

The Long Thin Life: If you are a middle-aged man, your life span will be 40 percent longer if you are one of the thinnest for your age rather than one of the heaviest. Further, you are 60 percent less apt to die of heart disease. That's the conclusion of a new study that tracked nineteen thousand Harvard alumni for twenty-seven years. Moreover, researchers found that over the years the heaviest men at any age had the greatest risk of death. The ideal weight for longevity in this study: around 20 percent below average. For example, a five-foot-ten-inch man who wants to live as long as possible should weigh no more than 157 pounds, 20 percent less than the average American male that height. (Note: The men were healthy nonsmokers, so their weight was not low because of smoking or disease.) Presumably the same general rules would apply to women, although similar studies have not been done.

Fewer Calories, Less Cancer: Shaving off calories had a startlingly quick and potent effect on the spread of precancerous cells in a recent study of overweight humans by researchers at Columbia University. Reducing daily calories by about one-third actually decreased the proliferation of precancerous cells in the colon by 40 percent. It's the first clear-cut evidence that restricting calories in humans can have an immediate antiaging anticancer effect.

If dietary restriction has the same effects in humans as it has in rodents, then human life span can be extended by at least 30 percent—which would give us an extra thirty to thirty-five years. But once we understand the mechanisms that control aging, we may find it possible to extend life span considerably

more, perhaps by 100 percent—which would give us
an extra one hundred years. —Dr. Edward Masoro,
physiologist and prominent calorie-restriction
researcher at the University of Texas Health Science
Center in San Antonio

―――――――

How Much Less Do You Have to Eat?

For caloric restriction to really kick in, says Dr. Walford,
you have to drop about 10 to 25 percent below your true
"ideal" weight or so-called personal "set-point," the weight
you tend to be when you are neither overeating nor undereating. It's usually the amount you weighed when you
were age twenty-five or thirty, if you were not overweight
then. If you are exceptionally lean, you need to reduce
calories by only about 10 percent. If you are obese, you
must cut calories by 25 to 30 percent, he says.

Probably any food and calorie restriction you make is
bound to help because it cuts down on production of pro-
aging free radicals. However, dropping to 30 to 40 percent
below normal, as in animal experiments, is too extreme to
be tolerated by most people. Researcher Ron Hart says
cutting calorie intake by 12 percent below normal delays
aging signs and adds some time to animals' life spans. He
thinks many Americans can let go of that many calories
without much hardship, as he has done.

How to Cut Calories to Stop Aging

Here is some advice on how to restrict calories to prolong
life, according to UCLA researcher Roy Walford, as noted
in his book *The 120-Year Diet*.

▲ Cut back calories gradually, so you lose bodily weight very slowly. Avoid extremely low-calorie crash diets. In animals, rapid caloric restriction did not prolong life. In fact, crash diets and prolonged fasting may shorten life. Envision a calorie-reduced diet that slowly takes off pounds over four to six years. As a start, an average-size man might try eating 2,000 calories per day, and a woman 1,800 calories per day of nutrient-dense foods. If you lose weight too fast, too slowly or not at all, adjust the food intake.

▲ The sooner you start a calorie-restricted diet after you are fully grown, the better. However, starting halfway through life should stretch your life about half as much as starting in young adulthood. Rodents who began on the diet at six months in some tests lived just as long as those who started the diet soon after birth. Starting even later in life should produce a proportionate benefit.

▲ Make every calorie count. Don't squander your youth on empty calories, such as sugar. Eat foods that are the most nutrient-dense—have the most nutrients and free radical compounds for the least calories. Of all foods, fruits and vegetables have the most antiaging substances for the least calories.

▲ Don't go on a restricted-calorie diet designed to postpone aging and age-related diseases before you are fully grown. Although caloric restriction from birth can stretch the life span of lab animals to the maximum, it also stunts their growth and sometimes brings an early death; severe caloric restriction could be disastrous for a growing child. This, of course, does not mean a growing child should be overweight; that transgression also can promote disease and premature aging in later life.

Caution: Severely calorie-restricted diets with the purpose of delaying aging and prolonging life are not appropriate for growing children, undernourished elderly persons or patients with serious diseases who may need more calories to thrive and survive.

Postscript: By studying animals on restricted diets, scientists hope to find certain biomarkers of aging that can then be modified in other ways, perhaps by shortcuts, such as specific nutrients or other supplements. For example, chromium supplements that increase insulin sensitivity may be one such nutrient that can partially mimic caloric restriction.

Get the Iron Out

▲ ▲ ▲

(Why You Need to Restrict Iron to Stop Aging)

Too much iron can make you old by fostering free radical attacks on cells. Don't routinely take iron supplements if you are an adult male or a woman past menopause.

Iron-poor blood. Tired blood. Iron-deficiency anemia. Such are the feared consequences of too little iron. But a greater danger for most men and older women is too much iron. Taking iron supplements and stuffing yourself with iron-rich foods can wreck your quest for the fountain of youth. High tissue stores of iron, especially past middle age, are more apt to make you sick and old than to keep you young and vital.

"Excess iron can be very dangerous," explains prominent researcher on aging Dr. Denham Harman of the University of Nebraska, because it facilitates free radical damage to cells. For example, iron helps change benign LDL cholesterol into the toxic type that wrecks arteries and makes hearts fail. Iron also aggravates the intensity of free radical reactions, furthering fierce free radical chain reactions that rip through many cells.

Heart Harm: Startling evidence from a 1992 Finnish study showed that men with the most iron in their blood were twice as likely to have heart attacks as men with the least iron-rich blood. (Iron was extra hazardous to men with high blood cholesterol.) A later Harvard study zeroed in on heme iron, found in meat and better absorbed than vegetable iron, as a culprit. Men with the most blood heme iron had 50 percent higher odds of heart attack than men with the least heme iron. Although the idea that iron might foster heart disease struck some as wacky, antiaging researchers were not surprised. Some had been preaching for more than a decade that iron is in cohoots with free radicals to do you in.

Although some studies have not identified iron as a culprit in heart disease, the role of iron and other metals in fostering free radical reactions provides compelling the-oretical reason to incriminate the metal in cell damage, aging and chronic diseases, including heart disease.

It makes sense that iron can be toxic, insists Jerome Sullivan, a pathologist at the Veteran Affairs Medical Center in Charleston, South Carolina, who first proposed the theory in 1981. He argues that the risk of heart attack rises in direct proportion to the amount of iron stored in the body. For example, he points out that men start having heart attacks in their twenties, after they are fully grown and begin to pile up iron in the blood and liver. In con-trast, premenopausal women who lose iron every month through menstruation are oddly protected from heart attacks. They succumb after menopause when menstrua-tion stops and iron builds up in the blood, although, of course, other factors such as estrogen may be involved.

According to Dr. Sullivan, there is no physiological reason whatever to encourage grown men or women after menopause to try to raise their bodily stores of iron. All you need is an adequate low-maintenance dose to keep things running smoothly, he says. Hoarding excess iron after that simply conspires with free radicals to make you age faster.

ANTIAGING SECRETS OF THE EXPERTS

Roy L. Walford, M.D., age seventy-one,
Professor of Pathology and Gerontology,
UCLA School of Medicine

Dr. Walford is one of the world's leading researchers in the field of aging, the man who applied his aging research to himself by embracing a restricted-calorie diet that he calls "the 120-year diet" to postpone aging and prolong life. On the diet he eats about 1,500 to 2,000 calories a day, about 30 percent fewer calories than normal—which has stretched life about 30 percent in virtually all animals tested.

Here's what Dr. Walford also takes every day to delay aging:

▲ Vitamin E—300 IU.
▲ Vitamin C—1,000 milligrams.
▲ Selenium—100 micrograms.
▲ Coenzyme Q-10—30 milligrams.

"By diet-restricting ourselves or finding the mechanism by which it works and applying it to humans, I think that people who are young may live to be 140 or 150 years old, and that means for the most part vigorous, functional years, not old age piled onto old age."

And Cancer, Too: If excess iron spurs free radical damage, it seems likely it would be incriminated in other aging diseases such as cancer. Sure enough. Iron is an overlooked cancer threat, finds Richard G. Stevens of the Pacific Northwest Laboratory in Richmond, Washington. His study of eight thousand persons noted that the higher the iron in blood, the greater the risk of cancer, especially bladder and esophageal cancer. Another 1994 study at the University of Illinois at Chicago showed that men and postmenopausal women with high blood iron were up to five times more apt to have precancerous colon polyps than those with lower blood iron levels. Polyps are tiny growths that can erupt into full-blown colon cancers.

Indeed, iron may help explain red meat's ability to stimulate colon cancer, regardless of the meat's fat content. Meat is rich in iron. In a Harvard study, women who ate about five ounces of beef, pork or lamb every day were 250 percent more apt to develop colon cancer than those who ate meat less than once a month. Fat was not totally responsible. The mysterious cancer-promoting factor in the meat could well be iron, say experts.

FIVE WAYS TO AVOID EXCESS IRON IF YOU ARE A MAN OR A WOMAN PAST MENOPAUSE

▲ Don't take individual iron supplements. Look for multivitamin-mineral tablets with low amounts of iron or no iron—certainly no more than 100 percent of the RDA. Beware that some multi formulas have alarmingly high amounts of iron—as much as 40 milligrams, more than 200 percent of the RDA.

▲ Cut down on animal foods. You absorb the heme iron in meat much more readily than the non-heme iron in vegetables such as beans and cereals. Red meat is particularly bad, says Emory University researcher Dr. Dean Jones, because it combines high iron with high fat—a perfect setting for the production of peroxides and free radicals. Indeed, a Harvard study by Dr. Alberto Ascherio found that men eating the most heme or red meat iron had a 43 percent higher risk of heart attack than those eating the least heme iron. It's riskier to get your iron from meat than from cereal, he says.

▲ Consume foods and beverages, such as tea, red wine and high-fiber bran and beans, that tend to block absorption of iron. This could be yet another reason tea drinkers tend to live longer, red wine drinkers seem to have less heart disease and fiber helps frustrate cancer. All three contain chemicals that limit iron's ability to foster cell-damaging interactions with free radicals.

▲ Beware of iron-fortified cereals. Some cereals such as Total and Product 19 contain 18 milligrams of iron per serving—100 percent of the RDA. Note: Such cereals are okay, indeed beneficial, for younger women and children who are often low in iron.

▲ If you are a man of any age or a woman past menopause, you might also help protect yourself by donating blood three times a year to deplete unwanted iron stores.

Caution: Menstruating women tend to lose iron regularly in blood flow and may need iron supplements.

Also, children and adolescents often do not get enough iron. The fact that extra dietary iron and iron supplements may be dangerous to men and post-menopausal women does not mean the same is true of younger women and children who lack iron. Adolescents, women of child-bearing age and children may need iron supplements to correct deficiencies.

The Danger Signs
of Needless Aging—
Antidotes and Remedies

▲   ▲   ▲   ▲   ▲   ▲   ▲

Falling apart, developing symptoms of disease, is so taken for granted as being a part of aging that we accept it as normal—part of our human fate programmed by nature and therefore inescapable. Most of it is not. Much of the change we attribute to normal aging is not preordained; it is accidental—a byproduct of our own ignorance or neglect—and can be avoided or remedied, within our individual genetic boundaries, by diet or supplements. Often, such "aging changes" stem from something as simple as a vitamin or antioxidant deficiency, and are amazingly reversible.

Pioneering researcher Bruce N. Ames, Ph.D., professor of biochemistry and molecular biology at the University of California at Berkeley, is blunt: "Aging appears to be in *most* part due to oxidants [free radicals] . . . Dietary antioxidants play a major role in minimizing this damage and most of the world's population is receiving inadequate amounts of them at a great cost to health."

Noted gerontologist Caleb Finch points out that some creatures never age biologically, although they grow old chronologically. Certain fish, for example, live to be one hundred without showing signs of aging, says Finch.

The amazing, unrecognized truth is: So much of aging is needless, and thus preventable and even reversible.

You are responsible in large part for your successful old age. Many of the aspects of being old that were considered due to the intrinsic aging process are really related to lifestyle. —Dr. John W. Rowe, head of the McArthur Foundation Research Network on Successful Aging and of New York's Mt. Sinai Hospital and School of Medicine

---

Don't Believe What
They Say About Senility!

▲　▲　▲

If your memory seems less sharp, you seem a little off-balance sometimes, or you notice other signs of "senility" in yourself or others, do not ignore it and do not palm it off as one of the tragedies of old age. It is often totally or partially reversible, and the sooner you try to arrest it, the better your odds of success.

It is sad, indeed, how many older people are condemned to a diagnosis of irreversible senility, their humanity and dignity taken from them, when their mental faculties could be preserved or retrieved by a few dollars' worth of vitamins and herbs or other simple dietary measures. Without question, we have the knowledge now to partially defeat humankind's most dreaded consequence of descent into old age—loss of mental faculties.

Your mind does not have to fail; your memory does not have to decline; you can take action early in life to help ward off later brain disintegration due to free radical damage, some experts suggest, and with certainty, you can prevent and often retrieve lost mental acuity due to a simple vitamin or other dietary deficiency or inadequate blood circulation.

We have come to realize that loss of mental capacity with age is not inevitable. The old idea that senility is a normal accompaniment of aging is simply wrong.
—Dr. Leonard Hayflick, gerontologist, University of California, San Francisco

---

How Free Radicals Can Destroy Your Brain and Antioxidants Can Save It

Your brain and memory can begin to malfunction because of accumulated free radical destruction of neurons, brain cells. And that's reason enough to keep those antioxidants flowing into your brain throughout a lifetime. The brain is particularly vulnerable because it's very fatty—rich in easily oxidized polyunsaturated fat; it's an oxygen factory, consuming one-fifth of all oxygen taken into the body; brain cells contain large amounts of iron that encourage free radical formation, and brain cells are fairly low in internally produced antioxidants, such as catalase and glutathione, to defend against free radical attacks. It's a hazardous mix.

Small wonder, then, that memory decline and degenerative brain disorders have been tied directly to free radical damage in brain cells.

The Alzheimer's Experiments: In new groundbreaking research, investigators at the University of Kentucky discovered evidence that in Alzheimer's disease, free radicals destroy normal brain cell function by binding to cells' protein and fat molecules. More remarkable, in lab tests the researchers were able to stop such Alzheimer's-like destruction in animal brain cells by adding antioxidants, including vitamin E. In short, they halted the process by which Alzheimer's destroys brain cells. This doesn't mean high doses of vitamin E will cure Alzheimer's, says Dr. William Markesbery, director of the University of Kentucky's Center on Aging, who has tested megadoses of vitamin E on Alzheimer's patients without much effect. But he thinks antioxidants taken early enough may prevent Alzheimer's or slow its progress. The University of Kentucky's Dr. Allan Butterfield, coauthor of the new study, says, "It could be a good idea" to take vitamin E regularly even in middle age, since it's not known to be harmful.

The Lou Gehrig's Discovery: MIT scientists have discovered a gene implicated in a form of Lou Gehrig's disease, a muscle-wasting disease also called amyotrophic lateral sclerosis or ALS. The gene apparently slashes levels of the antioxidant enzyme, superoxide dismutase, in half, allowing free radicals to kill neurons in the brain and spinal cord. Now under way are studies to determine if antioxidants, such as vitamins E and C, could block the free radical damage.

The Parkinson's Studies: It's not proof, but it's evidence. British researchers recently screened one hundred elderly people for signs of early Parkinson's disease. They found eight cases, six of them not previously diagnosed. They also discovered that a vitamin C deficiency seemed to help identify Parkinson's. A surprising 60 percent of those with a vitamin C deficiency had Parkinson's. Only 4 percent of the group without a vitamin C deficiency had the condition. Whether a lack of vitamin C contributes to causing Parkinson's is unknown. But researchers say there is strong evidence vitamin C can protect nerve cells from damage through antioxidant activity.

▲ Taking antioxidant vitamins early in life and as you age may erase mental deterioration and memory loss from your future.
▲ Getting antioxidants early in life could help prevent Alzheimer's disease, Parkinson's disease and Lou Gehrig's disease (ALS).
▲ Correcting a vitamin B deficiency could restore mental functioning and reverse "senility."

If I thought that you had [an early case of] Alz-heimer's today, I would tell you to take large doses of vitamin E and vitamin C. —Dr. William Markesbery, director of the University of Kentucky's Center on Aging

WHAT TO DO TO STOP MENTAL DETERIORATION

Get Enough Vitamin B12: A B12 deficiency is one of the most common causes of brain dysfunction with age. Surprisingly, at least 20 percent of people over age sixty and 40 percent over age eighty have a condition that, unless corrected, can trigger pseudo senility. It is called atrophic gastritis, and it simply means you no longer secrete enough stomach acid to absorb vitamin B12 and other neurologically critical vitamins, from food. Thus, gradually, without nourishment from B vitamins, the outer layer of nerve fibers deteriorate, creating neurological abnormalities. The first sign is often loss of balance, but symptoms also include loss of skin sensation, muscle weakness, incontinence, loss of vision, mood disturbances and even full-blown dementia and psychosis. And the longer the symptoms are allowed to persist unattended, the worse they become.

The fantastic news is that taking vitamin B12 pills usually prevents this mental deterioration, and B12 therapy, sometimes by injections, can reverse it if it is detected soon enough. A recent study of 143 patients with the problem by neurologist E. B. Healton and colleagues at Columbia-Presbyterian Medical Center found improvement in every single person after administration of high doses of B12. About half completely recovered their neurological functioning, and only 6 percent suffered long-term moderate or severe neurologic disability. The longer the duration of symptoms, the less the chance of full recovery, said Dr. Healton.

Try Folic Acid and B6: Unquestionably, a folic acid deficiency is strongly linked with brain dysfunction, depression and dementia, much research shows. A lack of folic acid and B6 is accompanied by a rise in blood homocysteine, a known brain toxin, and may be partly responsible for failing mental abilities during aging. (For doses and more details, see pages 76 and 79.)

Eat Tomatoes and Watermelon: Odd as it may seem, elderly women with high blood levels of an antioxidant called lycopene that is found almost exclusively in tomatoes, tomato products and watermelon are more mentally alert and better able to care for themselves than those with low blood lycopene, according to research at the University of Kentucky. It's probable that other antioxidants in fruits and vegetables may have similar effects in protecting aging brains. And, yes, it's expected the benefits would apply to aging men as well as women.

Try Ginkgo Extract: This herb supplement, extensively tested in Europe, stimulates blood circulation in the tiny vessels of the brain and has dramatically improved mental performance and memory in older persons. (For more details, see page 148.)

Give Vitamin E a Chance: Researchers suspect that vitamin E helps protect the fatty membranes in the brain from free radical damage leading to degenerative brain diseases and just plain forgetfulness and "senility." The vitamin may even help reverse failing mental abilities by restoring neurotransmitter receptor sites on brain cells so they can transmit critical brain signals as they did when you were younger, theorize Tufts University researchers. To get protective vitamin E, take supplements.

Take Garlic: Japanese experiments in animals indicate that garlic constituents protect neurons from damage and act as growth factors to stimulate the branching of brain cells. Giving aged garlic extract (Kyolic) to old animals restored some mental functions, including memory and problem-solving abilities.

Your Arteries Don't Need to Grow Old

▲　▲　▲

Hardening of the arteries is a supposed curse of old age. But it does not come from normal aging. Old animals rarely have it, nor do elderly people in certain populations. And it need not happen, although you do become more vulnerable with age to the hardening and thickening of artery walls known medically as atherosclerosis. Still, it's primarily a consequence of diet and lifestyle common in Western industrialized countries, where it is the number-one cause of aging, heart disease and death. The slow process of atherosclerosis begins as early as babyhood and progresses, gradually snuffing out life as arteries clog, triggering heart attacks and strokes. But it need not be an inevitable emblem of advanced age. You can intervene at any stage of life to slow it down, possibly even reverse it.

Exactly why arteries deteriorate is a complex biochemical puzzle. But scientists now recognize that free radicals and antioxidants, not surprisingly, have a big hand in it. Simply put, when, over many years, you regularly take in too many free radicals, as in animal fat and smoking, and too few antioxidants, as in vitamins and fruits and vegetables, your arteries become littered with debris embedded in artery walls—evidence of a prolonged free radical antioxidant battle in which free radicals consistently won. That truly characterizes an old artery.

Scientists suspect free radicals promote atherosclerosis in many ways by corrupting the normal activity of blood

components, such as leukocytes or white cells and fib-
rinogen, a clotting factor. But probably the most important
target of free radicals is LDL bad-type cholesterol.
According to a new theory, free radicals batter LDL fatty
molecules in vessel walls, turning them into rancid fat. This
crucial transformation of LDL is now thought to be the ini-
tiating step in the awful process of atherosclerosis. If this
LDL oxidation doesn't happen over and over, day in and
day out, your arteries may remain relatively young and
unclogged. Only after such cholesterol molecules become
rancid can they foment the complex process of building up
plaque to clog and stiffen arteries, the theory goes.

**The more easily oxidized your LDL cholesterol—
or put another way, the weaker your antioxidant
defenses—the more your arteries are aged and
wrecked by atherosclerosis.**

You can save your arteries from needless aging two
ways: One, keep free radical–generating fats and other
radicals from entering your blood. Two, keep a continual
flow of antioxidant soldiers in your blood to neutralize the
free radicals so they can't turn LDL rancid to destroy your
arteries. This stops the process of atherosclerosis at the
very instant of its genesis, no matter how old you are. Of
course, the earlier you start, the less aged your arteries
will become.

TRIPLE ANTIAGING HITS

Three of your best bets to ward off LDL oxidation and atherosclerosis are vitamin E, vitamin C and ubiquinol-10
(coenzyme Q-10), according to Balz Frei, Ph.D., free radical researcher in cardiovascular diseases at the Boston

VITAMIN E: ARTERY DETERGENT

A must for keeping arteries young and maybe even making them younger: at least 100 IU of vitamin E daily and preferably 400 IU. Studies show vitamin E helps keep arteries open after heart surgery (coronary bypass and angioplasty) and cuts odds of recurring heart attack by 40 to 50 percent and death by 20 percent. (See page 40 for more details.)

University School of Medicine. It's critical, he says, to buck up defenses both inside and outside the LDL molecule, and these three antioxidants work in concert. "Ubiquinol is the first line of defense," says Dr. Frei. Being fat-soluble, it gets inside the LDL molecule to fend off free radical attempts to oxidize the fat. By taking supplements or eating foods rich in coenzyme Q-10, you can boost its concentrations in LDL by five fold. But it is quickly exhausted in fighting off free radicals.

More reliable is fat-soluble vitamin E, which also fights off free radical oxidation from inside the LDL molecule. Vitamin C, on the other hand, is a sentry in the intracellular waters, keeping free radicals from breaking from the outside into LDL molecules. For best protection, then, you need good supplies of all three antioxidants, plus many others that can help out.

MAJOR WAYS TO KEEP ARTERIES YOUNG

▲ Restrict saturated animal fat, dairy fats, margarine and other trans fatty acids and foods high in omega-6 polyunsaturated fats such as corn oil and safflower oil. All encourage LDL toxicity and artery destruction.

▲ Restrict grilled, fried and broiled meat. They contain free radicals that attack artery walls.

▲ Take 100 IU and preferably 400 IU daily of vitamin E, a powerful deterrent to LDL oxidation. New studies show a minimum of 400 IU necessary for significant antioxidation effects.

▲ Eat foods high in ubiquinol-10 (coenzyme Q-10), such as sardines, and/or take coenzyme Q-10 supplements that block LDL oxidation.

▲ Eat fatty fish, such as salmon, mackerel, sardines and tuna fish, rich in omega-3 fatty acids, two or three times a week; they can inhibit oxidation and also act as an anticoagulant.

▲ Eat fruits and vegetables high in vitamin C and other antioxidant phenols, such as blueberries, oranges, red grapes, red grape juice and strawberries. Also take at least 500 milligrams daily of vitamin C, which protects LDL from oxidation.

▲ Drink tea. In tests it blocks LDL oxidation.

▲ Eat foods high in glutathione (fresh and frozen fruits and vegetables, such as avocado, asparagus and broccoli—see page 132) and/or take glutathione supplements. Glutathione cleanses food of oxidized fat hazard.

▲ Eat garlic. In tests it blocks LDL oxidation. Six hundred milligrams a day of garlic powder (six tablets of Kwai) reduced LDL oxidation 34 percent! Garlic also helps keep dangerous blood clots away.

▲ Use olive oil. In tests it helps block LDL oxidation. So do other monounsaturated fats in avocados and almonds.

▲ Go easy on sodium, which can stiffen and age arteries prematurely.

▲ If you drink alcoholic beverages, make it red wine in moderation—a glass or two a day— which can help prevent LDL oxidation and discourage blood clots; some protection persists in the bloodstream for almost twenty-four hours.

How to Stay Young at Heart

▲ ▲ ▲

Alas, your heart will grow steadily weaker as you age, losing some of its vital pumping functions, and possibly dissolving into heart failure—the number-one peril after age sixty-five. But you may be able to prevent and reverse some of the disintegrating function of your heart by protecting and strengthening the workings of tiny structures (mitochondria) inside cells that produce and transport the energy that keeps the heart strong and pumping.

It's a myth that your heart does not weaken as you get older. Several major studies suggest that heart function does not fizzle with age, that an older heart pumps just as well as a younger one. However, that may be true of a heart measured "at rest," but it's not true of ordinary aging hearts undergoing the normal stresses of life, according to Jeanne Y. Wei, M.D., director of the division on aging at Harvard Medical School.

Actually, the vital machinery of heart cells becomes increasingly damaged by free radical attacks as you age. Each heart cell, like other cells, has many tiny energy factories, called mitochondria, that are the "respiratory centers," the life force of cells, that keep them alive and functioning properly. But with age, large portions of the DNA of these mitochondria are literally chipped away. The weakened mitochondria then have to work harder; they require more oxygen. Consequently, the metabolic functioning of heart mitochondria declines by 40 percent in aged hearts, Dr. Wei says. In aged animals, the formation of vicious superoxide radicals in heart mitochondria surges 40 percent; mitochondria membranes become stiffened, stuffed with cholesterol and less efficient at transporting all-important ionized calcium that controls heart function. Microscopic photos of old animals' heart mitochondria show a scarred and tangled mess compared with those of young animals.

This relentless free radical damage to heart mitochondria over the years can lead to enlarged hearts, diastolic dysfunction (when blood flows back into the ventricle), reduction in blood flow, and congestive heart failure, exactly the symptoms that gradually beset aging populations. Half of all Americans have diastolic dysfunction after age eighty, and congestive heart failure is a growing epidemic, the number-one cause of hospitalization for Americans over age sixty-five, says Dr. Wei. Rates of congestive heart failure double every decade after age fifty.

"The old heart is simply less able to keep up. When there is something wrong with muscle function, let's say, or you have hypertension or a touch of arrhythmia, you can't generate enough energy to pump blood through the heart because you can't mobilize the machinery inside each of those heart cells to keep the muscles relaxing and contracting appropriately, so the heart will go into failure," explains Dr. Wei.

Worst of all, this cycle of damage to the heart mitochondria is self-perpetuating and accelerating. The more damaged they become over time, the less able they are to snuff out new damage, and it accumulates, picking up speed, causing more and more severe global heart dysfunction with age.

The big question: Can you delay this free radical–induced deterioration of the aging heart? Can you dispatch antioxidants to save the mitochondria and/or reduce the burden and reverse the dysfunction? Maybe. In one study, Dr. Wei gave aging animals oral doses of an amino acid called l-carnitine for two weeks. It did restore activity and function in the hearts of "middle-aged" rats, but not in very old ones. "Perhaps there is a window of time—after age fifty and before eighty, say, in which dysfunction is more easily reversed," says Dr. Wei.

SOME WAYS TO SAVE AND REVIVE AN AGING HEART

Get Lots of Antioxidant Vitamins: The major antioxidant vitamins—vitamin E, vitamin C and beta carotene, as well as others—may all help prevent massive free radical damage to mitochondria or power factories in heart cells. Such damage in heart mitochondria is especially risky because it means snuffing out power, bringing an energy shutdown in the very organ without which life ceases. Such free radical damage can slash power output in cell mitochondria as much as 80 percent, say experts, seriously disrupting heart functions. As insurance to keep heart mitochondria burning efficiently, take a multiple-vitamin pill as well as extra vitamin E, vitamin C, beta carotene, selenium and magnesium. Also eat lots of antioxidant-packed fruits and vegetables.

Try Coenzyme Q-10: Much research, including nine double-blind controlled studies, documents that coenzyme Q-10 restores critical energy production to heart mitochondria, dramatically improving heart function and often rescuing people from debilitating and potentially deadly heart failure. CoQ-10, as it is called, is a natural substance that the body produces in smaller quantities as we age. It has been synthesized and is sold as a supplement. CoQ-10 is a strong antioxidant that may help prevent as well as reverse the cumulative effects of years of cellular damage in an aging heart. (For more details, see page 138.)

Consider Carnitine: This is an amino acid produced by your body; you also get some by eating meat and dairy products, and you can get it as a supplement in health food stores. A great deal of evidence finds that l-carnitine is essential to optimal functioning of heart mitochondria. It can improve stress tolerance in damaged heart muscle in humans, research also shows. Research by Harvard's Dr. Wei also found that 40 percent of rats given carnitine two-thirds of the way through life lived three months longer than non–carnitine-fed rats. Moreover, the hearts of the carnitine-fed rats were stronger and the animals did distinctly better on mental tests.

Texas researcher and cardiologist Peter Langsjoen sometimes has patients with congestive heart failure take l-carnitine along with coenzyme Q-10. Adding 1,000 milligrams of l-carnitine (250 milligrams four times a day) in some cases is more effective than coQ-10 alone in restoring heart function, he finds. A dosage of 10 to 30 milligrams of l-carnitine per kilogram (2.2 pounds) of body weight has been suggested as an antiaging human dose, according to UCLA's Roy Walford. That would be at least 600 milligrams daily for a 125-pound woman and 800 milligrams for a 170-pound man. New York physician Stephen DeFelice takes 1,000 milligrams daily to help retard aging. L-carnitine may be an antiaging agent, Dr. Walford says, but it is still unclear.

Restrict Meat: Studies at the National Institutes of Health find severe damage to the heart muscle of animals fed cooked meats high in heterocyclic amines—HCAs—chemicals formed when you cook meat, especially at high temperatures. (See page 219.)

Eat Fish: The omega-3 fatty acids in fish can improve heart function by helping prevent arrhythmias, irregular heartbeats that can trigger sudden death. Fish high in such fatty acids are salmon, mackerel, sardines, herring and tuna.

The Aging Toxin It's Easy to Abolish

▲ ▲ ▲

You definitely don't want high homocysteine in your blood. Yet it creeps up with age, along with worsening vitamin B deficiencies, and afflicts some 30 to 40 percent of older adults. It turns millions of Americans into unwitting victims of needless aging by blocking blood vessels, precipitating heart attacks and strokes. You could well be one, since hardly anyone is aware of homocysteine's threat or what it is. Homocysteine is a type of amino acid in the blood that, like cholesterol, becomes oxidized and releases floods of the vicious free radical superoxide. Homocysteine, in fact, may be more pernicious than cholesterol at destroying your arteries. Yet it is far easier to correct.

Artery Poison: High blood levels of homocysteine triple your chances of heart attack and double your risk of blockage of the carotid (neck and head) arteries, a common cause of stroke, according to new research at Harvard and Tufts. Even a modest blockage of such carotid arteries also ups your odds of heart attack by 700 percent, according to a Finnish study. If you have heart disease, it's probable that your blood homocysteine is about one-third higher than that of people without heart disease. Jacques Genest, M.D., and colleagues at the Montreal Heart Institute found that 44 percent of a group of women and 18 percent of a group of men with heart disease had abnormally high levels of homocysteine. An Irish study noted that 30 percent of middle-aged subjects under age fifty-five with clogged arteries had high homo-cysteine. Yet all those with clear, open arteries had normal homocysteine. Another fact: Children born with a genetic defect, leaving them with super-high homocys-teine, often die in their teens or early twenties of severe cardiovascular disease.

Homocysteine ages arteries three ways, says Dr. Genest: It directly attacks the walls of blood vessels, injuring cells and inciting vessels to constrict. It activates factors that cause blood clotting. It stimulates growth of smooth muscle cells that line arteries, promoting buildup of plaque.

At least 10 percent of all heart attacks, or 150,000 every year, are tied to high homocysteine levels.
—Harvard researcher Meir J. Stampfer

Brain Poison: Abnormally high homocysteine also poi-sons your mood and mental acuity. By measuring homo-cysteine levels, scientists can predict depression as well as mental impairment, such as declines in memory, concen-tration and thinking abilities that have routinely been blamed on aging. For example, Dr. Iris Bell, an assistant professor of psychiatry at the University of Arizona, has found that depressed elderly patients with high homocys-teine levels scored lower on mental tests than did young depressed patients. The afflicted elderly showed a greater loss of memory and ability to learn, indicating a decline in brain function.

Dr. Bell and colleagues speculate that excess homocys-teine damages blood vessels in the brain the same way it does heart arteries. Also, homocysteine converts to another substance that in excess can cause brain cells to self-

ANTIAGING SECRETS OF THE EXPERTS

Stephen DeFelice, M.D.
Chairman of the Foundation for
Innovation in Medicine

Dr. DeFelice is a pioneering advocate in the use of natural substances he calls "nutraceuticals," including vitamins, minerals and other supplements, to prevent and treat the diseases of aging.

Here's what Dr. DeFelice takes daily:

▲ Vitamin E—200 IU.
▲ Vitamin C—300 milligrams.
▲ L-carnitine—1,000 milligrams.
▲ Magnesium chloride—350 milligrams.

destruct, she says. "The fact that homocysteine is a neurotoxin really emphasizes the importance of keeping its levels low," says Dr. Jeffrey Blumberg at Tufts Human Nutrition Research Center on Aging.

THE CURE IS QUICK, CHEAP AND SAFE

What's the reason for dangerously high homocysteine? It's simple: low blood levels of B vitamins—namely folic acid, B6 and to a lesser extent B 12. Although homocysteine has been recognized as a predictor of artery clogging and heart disease for about a quarter century, only recently have researchers discovered that high homocysteine occurs mostly in people lacking these B vitamins. According to

Harvard research, about two-thirds of high homocysteine is linked to low levels of folic acid, B6 and/or B12. Even borderline deficiencies of these vitamins can cause elevated homocysteine. Moreover, low vitamin B levels are a dead giveaway for blocked arteries.

Now the astonishingly good news: You can bring down homocysteine remarkably fast by taking folic acid, B6 and B12. The vitamins are necessary to help metabolize—break down—homocysteine so it can be destroyed. When there is not enough of these B vitamins in the blood to dispose of the homocysteine, it builds up and becomes hazardous.

If you have high homocysteine, you're more apt to have blocked arteries, heart disease and vitamin B deficiencies. Taking B vitamins quickly reduces homocysteine, thus lowering your risk of clogged arteries, heart attacks and strokes.

FOOD OR PILLS?

Nobody is yet sure the dose of B vitamins it takes to control homocysteine. If you have high homocysteine, pioneer researcher Dr. Rene Malinow, professor of medicine at the Oregon Health Sciences University, favors taking 1,000 to 5,000 micrograms a day of folic acid and 10 to 50 milligrams of B6 supplements to suppress the hazard. Dr. Malinow himself takes 1,000 daily micrograms of folic acid as a preventive. Dr. Jacob Selhub, homocysteine researcher at the U.S. Department of Agriculture's Human Nutrition Research Center on Aging at Tufts University, says his research finds intakes of 350 micrograms of folic acid and 2 to 2.5 milligrams of B6 daily enough to keep homocysteine at low levels in most people.

That means you could curb homocysteine by the

amounts of folic acid in a multiple vitamin or by eating folic acid–rich foods, for 350 micrograms can be obtained in the daily diet. Still, depending entirely on food may be risky; most Americans average only 235 micrograms daily; elderly people are worse off. Also, only half the folic acid in most foods is absorbed. A recent study by South African authority J. B. Ubbink found that the folic acid in food did not suppress high homocysteine in about two-thirds of elderly subjects.

In his study of heart patients with high homocysteine, Dr. Genest initially gave 2.5 to 5 daily milligrams of folic acid (2,500 to 5,000 micrograms). If that did not lower homocysteine, he added 50 milligrams of B6. He found that these doses of the two vitamins depressed homocysteine about 50 percent in 90 percent of the patients within two weeks. He calls such doses "very safe and effective."

Which of the B vitamins is most powerful at reducing homocysteine? Folic acid, say experts, followed by B6 and B12. In one Tufts study, adequate doses of all three were needed to keep homocysteine under control.

Can You Be Tested for High Homocysteine? Doctors do not routinely test for homocysteine; the tests are still used mostly for research, but many experts think they will soon become standard in preventing, diagnosing and treating heart disease.

How to Ward Off Dangerous Homocysteine

▲ Eat foods high in folic acid and B6. Sources of folic acid are spinach, collard greens, beet greens, legumes and nuts. Good sources of B6 are seafood, whole grains, bananas, nuts and poultry.

▲ Take vitamin B pills: folic acid, B6 and B12. You can get the basic amounts of each in a multiple vitamin, which seems enough in preventing rises in homocysteine. Higher doses, such as 1,000 micrograms of folic acid and 10 milligrams of vitamin B6, require separate tablets and may be needed to lower excessively high homocysteine if you have heart disease. Such doses are not toxic; however, if you take one, you should take all three—folic acid, B6 and B12—for maximum protection (one study found you needed higher than average levels of all three to achieve the lowest homocysteine levels) and to prevent a dangerous imbalance.

Note: When you discontinue the vitamins, homocysteine tends to shoot back up. In one study, homocysteine rose back up to abnormally high levels in two-thirds of the subjects within eighteen weeks of discontinuing their B vitamins.

Since there's no way to know if you have abnormally high homocysteine, it makes sense to take modest doses of folic acid, B6 and B12 as anti-aging insurance. They may help blot out heart disease and mental impairment related to undetected insufficiency of the B vitamins.

Caution: *If you have heart disease, consult your physician before taking high doses of B vitamins to try to correct high homocysteine.*

Fact: Your homocysteine becomes elevated when you are merely borderline deficient in folic acid or B6. High homocysteine is a good biomarker of a vitamin B6 and folic acid deficiency.

THE INCREDIBLE FIX

Here are the daily vitamin B doses a group of international experts recommends to reduce and normalize high homocysteine in those with heart disease, according to Dr. M. Rene Malinow, professor of medicine at Oregon Health Sciences University:

Folate (folic acid)—1 to 5 milligrams.
B6—10 to 50 milligrams.
B12—up to 1,000 micrograms.

Your Failing Immunity Is Reversible!

▲　▲　▲

Deteriorating immunity is one of the most prominent hallmarks of aging. Indeed, your immune functions start slipping away by age thirty, starting with a decline in the number and activity of your T-cells that fight off viruses and tumor cells and help other white cells fend off invasions of bacteria and other dangerous elements. Researchers at Tufts University have shown that an immune suppressor in the blood called prostaglandin E2 rises steadily with age, helping explain why the older you get, the more apt you are to have infections and cancer.

Your immune functioning even predicts how long you will live and whether you develop cancer. One study of healthy people over age sixty found that those with less vigorous immune systems were twice as apt to die of any cause, and about 30 percent more apt to get cancer.

But the amazing truth is that so much of this "aging" is needless and reversible! And it is reversible in many cases by simply taking modest to high doses of certain vitamins and minerals, according to impressive new research. Vitamins rev up immune functions at any age, including childhood. Even the very elderly can regain immune functions, Tufts researchers have found.

It's undeniable. You simply don't need to tolerate ever-weakening immune functions. Faltering immunity is one of the prime biomarkers of aging. That it can be easily, safely and cheaply reversed is one of the exciting and generally unappreciated discoveries of modern medicine.

If you do nothing else to boost immunity, take a multivitamin pill every day, the kind you can buy at any drugstore. For more antiaging power, try separate vitamin E and vitamin C supplements.

How to Preserve and Rejuvenate Immunity

Take a Multivitamin Mineral Pill: It seems too amazing to be true. But solid evidence shows that just taking a single drugstore multivitamin-mineral pill every day can dramatically improve immune system capabilities to fight off infections as well as cancer. In one double-blind study of sixty healthy men and women aged fifty-nine to eighty-five, Dr. John D. Bogden and colleagues at the University of Medicine and Dentistry of New Jersey found that taking Theragran-M, an over-the-counter supplement of twenty-four vitamins and minerals, improved immune responses dramatically. Indeed, after a year, the vigor of immune responses soared an astonishing 64 percent! Specifically, vitamin takers produced more all-important T-lymphocyte cells (white blood cells) as well as antibodies and other substances that spur the immune system to spring into action to fight infections.

Even older people who consume pretty good diets experience enhanced immunity by taking a multivitamin supplement. —Dr. John D. Bogden, University of Medicine and Dentistry of New Jersey

---

Another groundbreaking study that opened the eyes of mainstream medicine to the infection-fighting and immunity-bolstering powers of vitamins was done by leading immunologist Ranjit Kumar Chandra, of Memorial University of Newfoundland. He presented compelling evidence showing that taking modest doses of vitamins and minerals for a year squelched infections in a group of ninety-six healthy elderly men and women. In fact, vitamin takers had only half as many days of debilitating infectious illness as those taking a dummy pill. The special formulation of eighteen vitamins and minerals triggered broad improvement in the number of T-cells, lymphocyte response, interleukin-2 production, IL-2 receptor release, natural killer cell activity and antibody response to the influenza vaccine. All the doses were moderate, about what you would find in a typical multivitamin tablet, except for higher doses of antioxidant beta carotene (16 milligrams) and vitamin E (44 milligrams). Dr. Chandra attributed the strongest immune system improvement to vitamin A, beta carotene, zinc and vitamin E.

Up to one-third of the subjects had unknown vitamin and trace mineral deficiencies that apparently suppressed immune functioning, said Dr. Chandra, and correcting them restored immune functioning.

Take Extra Vitamin E: To give immune functioning another powerful jumpstart, you need vitamin E supplements. "It has a tremendous effect," raves Tufts researcher Mohsen Meydani. "If everyone got vitamin E through the years, immune functioning simply would not decline the way it does now with age." Vitamin E supplements both preserve immunity as you age and rejuvenate it when you are old, well into your eighties. In tests, Dr. Mohsen Meydani and his wife, Dr. Simin Meydani, have found that taking vitamin E (only 400 IU daily for six months) preserves and/or rejuvenates the weakened immune functioning in both the young and the old—even though they don't lack vitamin E to begin with. In other words, vitamin E has super immune-elevating powers above simply correcting deficiencies. The vitamin actually retards aging changes that result in declining immune functioning. And if your immune system is already faltering, vitamin E doses will bring it back to youthful activity. The Meydanis believe one important way vitamin E works is by suppressing production of prostaglandin E2, a hormonelike substance that ordinarily surges as you age and helps wreck immune functioning.

Vitamin E also keeps viruses from breaking out and replicating, according to U.S. Department of Agriculture studies.

Take Vitamin B6: If you lack vitamin B6, your immune system malfunctions. Your body can't produce enough interleukin-2 and lymphocytes to fight off infections, as well as cancer and arthritis. Tufts researchers found that without vitamin B6, immune functioning sank. But when subjects got B6 supplements for three weeks (1.9 milligrams per day for women and 2.88 milligrams per day for men), immunity bounced up to normal in most individuals. The need for B6 increases after age forty or so, and you begin to need amounts from 20 to 45 percent above the current recommended doses to prevent or delay age-related changes in the immune system.

Take Zinc: Be sure to get enough zinc to keep your thymus gland from wasting away and killing your immune responses. (See page 92.) You can often get some immune-protecting zinc (15 milligrams) in a multiple-vitamin mineral pill.

Take Vitamin C: Vitamin C increases production of white blood cells to fight off infections. Further, vitamin C boosts blood levels of glutathione, critical for proper immune functioning. Five hundred milligrams daily of vitamin C may keep immunity high; if you already have an infection, such as the flu or a cold, much higher doses (several thousand milligrams daily) are needed to relieve symptoms.

Get Enough Selenium: A lack of selenium can turn viruses from benign to very ugly, able to trigger mechanisms that allow them to replicate and cause illnesses. There's evidence selenium also boosts immunity to cancer. Eating selenium-rich food and/or taking supplements with selenium or a separate pill (100 to 200 micrograms) daily is enough, say experts. (See page 117.) Beware: Selenium in high doses can be toxic.

Eat Yogurt: Yogurt's bacterial cultures boost immune functioning. Eating a couple of cups of ordinary yogurt a day for a year raised infection-fighting gamma interferon in the blood of old and young people 500 percent, according to research by immunology professor Georges Halpern, M.D., at the University of California at Davis. In another study, he found that people who ate a cup of yogurt a day for a year had 25 percent fewer colds compared with non–yogurt eaters. The yogurt had live active cultures of *Bulgaricus lactobacillus* and *Streptococcus thermophilus,* which is standard for yogurt sold in the United States.

An Avoidable Aging Bombshell

▲ ▲ ▲

You may have an unknown aging promoter in your blood-stream that gets out of hand sometime in midlife and begins silently attacking your arteries, draining your energy, raising your blood pressure, hustling you toward diabetes and even fertilizing the growth of tumors that may be lurking in your body. The substance is the hormone insulin—vital to life in normal amounts, but malevolent and deadly in excess. It grows bold with age.

Insulin is everybody's potential nemesis. It's impossible to hold on to your youth if excesses of insulin are raging through your bloodstream. Luckily, however, you can keep a lid on insulin, for its misbehavior is largely another sign of needless aging. If you don't normalize insulin, you can face diabetes, artery clogging, severe heart disease, and premature death.

Some time after age thirty-five, especially if you typically gain weight as you get older, insulin levels in your blood are likely to rise, along with blood sugar (glucose) levels. And that's bad news. Insulin is the hormone that gets out of whack, triggering diabetes. But a string of incredible new evidence also identifies insulin as a central, underlying cause of a whole constellation of conditions that strike with aging. An oversupply of insulin has been indicted as a conspirator in high blood sugar, high cholesterol, high blood pressure, high triglycerides (another dangerous blood fat) and low good-type HDL cholesterol. Some experts frankly blame excesses of insulin—or "hyperinsulinemia"—for much of our epidemic of heart disease. Daniel W. Foster, M.D., University of Texas Southwestern Medical Center, has branded a malfunction of insulin "a secret killer."

Leading gerontologist and diabetes expert Gerald Reaven, M.D., at Stanford University, agrees, saying that millions of Americans, who have no warning signs, are insulin's unwitting victims-to-be, exceedingly vulnerable to heart disease and diabetes. Dr. Reaven documented that about 25 percent of all seemingly normal, healthy nondiabetic older Americans have so-called insulin resistance. That means cells won't let insulin do its job of ushering sugar (glucose) into cells so it can be converted to energy. Consequently, blood levels of both sugar and insulin may soar; the pancreas may even frantically churn out more insulin to try to keep blood sugar normal. But insulin resistance doesn't happen just because you're aging, declares Dr. Reaven. You don't have to get it. And if you do have it, you can correct it before it does irreversible damage.

How Too Much Insulin Can Make You Old

Destroys Arteries: Insulin triggers artery clogging by stimulating the growth of smooth muscle cells on artery walls. Such cell proliferation is essential to the progression of atherosclerosis in which plaque builds up, narrowing arteries and cutting down on blood flow. Insulin also interferes with the clot-dissolving system by stimulating high levels of plasminogen activator inhibitor-1. Thus, a clot is more apt to form, blocking the artery.

Raises Bad Cholesterol: Insulin revs up the liver's production of LDL bad-type cholesterol, the type that eventually gets plastered into artery walls. Additionally, people with excessive insulin and insulin resistance are more apt to have smaller, denser LDL particles. These are the worst, most apt to become oxidized, contributing to artery clogging. Individuals with high concentrations of such LDL particles are three times more apt to have a heart attack, according to Dr. Reaven.

Raises Triglycerides: No question, excessive insulin is a primary cause of high triglycerides, a blood fat once thought relatively harmless, but now considered dangerous. As triglycerides rise, unfortunately, levels of good-type HDL cholesterol fall, dramatically increasing your risk of heart disease. HDL molecules transport bad-type LDL cholesterol to the liver for destruction. Therefore, you want vast armies of these carriers in your blood.

Raises Blood Pressure: If you have high blood pressure, chances are fifty-fifty that you also are insulin-resistant and have excessive malfunctioning insulin in your blood. How insulin might help regulate blood pressure is unclear and controversial. One theory is that insulin affects the regulation of the kidneys and/or the nervous system, causing blood vessels to constrict and raise pressure.

Triggers Diabetes: An often constant companion of excessive insulin is excessive blood glucose—or glucose intolerance, possibly foreshadowing diabetes. "Glucose intolerance today, diabetes tomorrow" is how many researchers see it. This doesn't mean that everybody with glucose intolerance will develop diabetes. But nobody develops diabetes who does not have glucose intolerance.

Stimulates Cancer Growth: Insulin has been shown to be a growth promoter of malignant cells.

How to Control Aging by Controlling Insulin

Watch the Sugar: Don't eat lots of sugar and carbohydrates. The more sugar or carbohydrates you take in, the more of it you must process, and that requires more insulin. All sugars can equally boost insulin needs—ordinary table sugar, sugar in cakes and cookies, as well as fructose in fruit and fruit juices and honey.

Don't Eat Bad Fat: Eating fat that is rapidly oxidized triggers the release of insulin and buildup of glucose in the blood. The most diabolic are polyunsaturated fats, such as corn oil, and regular safflower and sunflower seed oils that infuse your blood with free radical peroxides. If you don't have enough antioxidants to mop them up, the radicals shut down an enzyme that metabolizes sugar. Thus glucose blood levels rise, and the body pours out more insulin in attempts to handle the sugar.

The only safe fat is monounsaturated fat, as in olive oil, canola oil, avocados and nuts, which is not easily oxidized; thus it does not set in motion the cascade of events leading to excessive insulin.

Take Chromium: It's a must. Take 200 micrograms of organic chromium, such as picolinate or GTF trivalent, daily to keep insulin at normal levels and working efficiently. If you lack chromium, your body is apt to compensate by pouring out more insulin. As USDA researcher Dr. Richard Anderson says: "Chromium makes insulin more efficient so you need less to do the job." He advises young as well as older adults to take chromium. It's not too early to start as a teenager, he says. (See page 81.)

Lose Weight If You Are Overweight: "The heavier you are and the less active you are, the more insulin resistant you will be, no matter what your genetic makeup," says Dr. Reaven. Simply being 20 percent overweight (the definition of obese) can bring on insulin resistance. Being 40 percent over ideal weight suppresses insulin's ability to process sugar by 30 to 40 percent. You're more apt to have insulin resistance if your weight is in the upper body—the apple shape instead of the pear shape. You don't have to be overweight to have an insulin problem, but taking off pounds does strikingly stimulate normal insulin activity and banish some of the excesses.

Take Vitamin E: It can spur insulin activity. When a group of healthy elderly Italians took 900 milligrams of vitamin E a day, their insulin's ability to do its job of disposing of blood sugar more than doubled. The researchers at the University of Naples believe vitamin E protected the integrity of the membranes from oxidative free radical damage, making cells better able to use insulin in transporting glucose. In short, vitamin E reversed age-related insulin resistance and weak insulin activity. Note: Lower doses of E will probably also work.

A Tad of Alcohol: A little drinking stimulates your insulin activity, so you need less of it to process sugar. Stanford's Dr. Reaven found that light to moderate drinkers (one or two drinks a day) had lower blood sugar, and about 55 percent less insulin, as well as higher HDL cholesterol, than nondrinkers.

Spice Things Up: Surprisingly, cinnamon, cloves, turmeric and bay leaves stimulate insulin efficiency, meaning your body gets by with less of the hormone.

Forget Three Square: Grazing is better than chowing down three times daily. That's because big meals send your insulin and blood sugar up more steeply. In a group of Type II diabetics, insulin levels spurted up much higher after they had eaten two large meals than after they had eaten six small meals. Also, their blood sugar levels did a yo-yo, rising 84 percent from the lowest level. In another study of nondiabetic women, eating nine small meals a day instead of three big ones had similar insulin benefits; their cholesterol also fell 6.5 percent.

You get much healthier blood sugar and insulin levels from having three small meals and three snacks throughout the day. —Dr. Aaron Vinik, director of the Diabetes Research Institute in Norfolk, Virginia

---

Cancer: You Can
Grow Old Without It

▲ ▲ ▲

Undeniably, cancer comes with age. Eighty percent of all cancers happen after age sixty-five, and by the end of life about one-third of us will be stricken by cancer. But cancer is not due to aging itself. It strikes later in life because longevity provides cancer a longer incubation period in which to develop. Cancer is not an overnight phenomenon like an infection; it is a long, slow process that happens over twenty, thirty, forty years, as cells are bombarded by free radicals, causing initial mutations in genetic DNA, followed by years of tiny encouragements to grow into a tumor and then to spread to other tissues in the body. Cancer is a long time coming. A cancer discovered today is the result of free radical catastrophes that began occurring several decades ago and are still piling up.

Gino Cortopassi and colleagues at the University of Southern California, Los Angeles, have documented the accelerating toll that time imposes on cells. Mutations are thirteen times more frequent in the blood cells and forty times more frequent in the spleen cells of people over age sixty compared with those under age twenty, he found. Such accumulation of mutations can eventually turn genes on or off over time, triggering cancer, he says. Thus, cancer is one more random consequence of weakened cell resistance to accumulated radical damage. But if you can impede this buildup of cell mutations, you can put a powerful roadblock in the path of cancer.

You don't get cancer because you age. You get cancer because, by living longer, you give cell mutations time to build up, inciting cancer, among other catastrophes. By bucking up your cells' declining defenses to damage, you may delay cancer or postpone it for a lifetime. Not everyone gets cancer, and you can grow old without it.

To be sure, your cancer odds are influenced by genetics, lifestyle and environment and subtle interactions among them. But any barriers you erect at any instant of any developmental stage can help thwart cancer's journey. The most powerful deterrents within your control are antioxidant defenses. Even after you have precancerous signs of cancer or cancer itself, antioxidants may increase your odds of survival. Some experts believe we could escape the vast majority of cancers by eating the right diet, taking in lots of antioxidants and not smoking.

What you need to do is keep your cells from becoming so heavily damaged that genes (called oncogenes) are compelled to start the wild proliferation of cells that add up to cancer. Curb as much damage as possible by ridding yourself of exposure to free radicals, such as cigarette smoke, that irreparably change the genetic code of cells, making them malignant. At the same time, try to block your cells' declining resistance, rendering them less able to fight off cancer-inspiring free radical damage.

VITAMIN BREAKTHROUGHS

At the very least, be sure you get enough antioxidant vitamins to maintain a minimal cellular defense. The exciting fact is that there is impeccable, concrete proof that vitamin-mineral supplements can prevent human cancers, as shown

ANTIAGING SECRETS OF THE EXPERTS

Jeffrey Blumberg, Ph.D., age forty-six
Associate Director, U.S.D.A. Human Nutrition
Research Center on Aging at Tufts University

Dr. Blumberg is a leading advocate of antioxidant supplements to combat premature aging.
Here's what he takes every day:

- ▲ Vitamin E—400 IU.
- ▲ Vitamin C—250 to 1,000 milligrams.
- ▲ Beta carotene—15 milligrams (25,000 IU).
- ▲ A multivitamin-mineral formula with 100 to 200 percent of the RDA for various vitamins and minerals.

"If you look at risk versus benefit, what we're talking about is some potential benefit and zero risk, and the balance turns out to be in favor of antioxidant supplements."

in a groundbreaking 1993 study by the U.S. National Cancer Institute in a rural Chinese population. For five years, a group of Chinese took daily doses of antioxidant beta carotene, vitamin E and selenium. Their cancer deaths dropped 13 percent in that incredibly short time. Esophageal cancer deaths fell 4 percent, stomach cancer deaths, 21 percent. Rates of all other cancers decreased 20 percent. Amazingly, the research team, headed by NCI's William Blot, reported that cancer deaths began to drop within one to two years after the supplements were started. Stroke rates also declined. The supplement doses were low and may have simply corrected deficiencies. Regardless, the point is, the antioxidants did combat cancer, presumably by guarding cells from free radical damage.

Even more startling, vitamin megadoses can help fight existing cancer. In a recent study by Dr. Donald Lamm, head of urology at West Virginia University in Morgantown, high-dose vitamin supplements dramatically cut the recurrence of bladder cancer and nearly doubled the survival time of patients.

But a burning question is: How late can antioxidants intervene to stop cancer? Can you continue to smoke, for example, and expect antioxidants to save you? No. A recent Finnish study found that taking 20 milligrams of beta carotene and 50 IU of vitamin E daily did not prevent lung cancer in those who had smoked two packs a day for thirty years and continued to smoke.

ANTIAGING STRATEGY: HOW TO SAY NO TO CANCER

▲ Eat five or more servings of fruits and vegetables a day. The evidence is overwhelming that fruits and vegetables contain powerful agents that turn off and slow down cancer. About two hundred studies find that eating fruits and vegetables cuts the risk of cancer, even among the elderly, by about 50 percent.

▲ Drink tea; it's full of antioxidants, keeps laboratory animals free of cancer and is linked to lower risk of certain cancers in humans. (This means "real" tea, not herbal teas, which are not known to have the same antioxidant powers as ordinary black, green and oolong tea.)

▲ Restrict red meat. It's linked to cancers of the colon, breast and prostate.

▲ Restrict saturated animal fat. It promotes ovarian cancer and fatal breast cancer and possibly other cancers.

▲ Go easy on alcohol. More than a drink a day raises the risk of breast cancer in women. Excessive beer is a rectal cancer threat. Alcohol promotes some types of colon cancer and is a big cause of esophageal cancer.

▲ Eat more soybean protein in soy flour, soy milk, tempeh, tofu and the whole bean itself. Soybeans are full of anticancer agents and appear to specifically help prevent breast and prostate cancer.

▲ Take vitamins and minerals, at least a one-a-day vitamin-mineral pill to bring cellular defenses up to a minimal status. Then if you want some extra insurance, do as many cancer researchers do: Add daily vitamin C (500 to 2,000 milligrams), vitamin E (400 IU) and beta carotene (10 to 20 milligrams). Consider other supplements, such as garlic and selenium, at doses discussed in this book.

▲ If you smoke, quit.

The Mythology of Rising Blood Pressure

▲ ▲ ▲

Sure, your blood pressure is likely to rise as you get older. According to one study, systolic blood pressure (upper number) jumps an average 15 points between ages twenty-five and fifty-five. Such age-related rises are typical in industrialized countries, such as the United States. It's even worse in Japan. But the important fact is that blood pressure does not universally go up in people of all cultures—particularly not in less developed countries. Thus, soaring blood pressure, an epidemic in this country, is not an inevitable phenomenon of aging. It, like many chronic diseases, is another sign of needless aging that you can control to some extent, depending on genetic susceptibility.

Once again, it's often a case of too many free radicals versus too few antioxidants. New evidence finds high blood pressure at least in part a free radical–created disease that may be curbed by antioxidants, along with other dietary factors, such as sodium, calcium, alcohol and weight. One theory: Increased free radical generation blocks production of nitric oxide and prostacyclin, both blood vessel relaxants that help keep blood pressure down.

Eating more antioxidants in fruits and vegetables and taking antioxidant supplements, especially vitamin C, can stave off rising blood pressure.

SO BRING ON THE ANTIOXIDANTS

Eating more antioxidants throughout your life can help defeat rising blood pressure as you age. In one study, noted authority Jeremiah Stamler of Northwestern University Medical School in Chicago found that the blood pressure of men who ate the most vitamin C and beta carotene over ten years did not rise as much as that of those eating the least of such vitamins. The difference, though small, translates into a 6 percent reduction in deaths from stroke, 4 percent from heart disease and 3 percent from all causes.

Vitamin C appears particularly potent in keeping blood pressure down, according to overwhelming evidence. Numerous studies show that high blood pressure is highest among people who eat the least vitamin C. Tufts researchers, for example, found that people who failed to get the daily vitamin C in just one orange (70 milligrams) averaged 11 points higher systolic (upper number) and 6 points higher diastolic pressure than those eating more vitamin C. In general, low blood levels of vitamin C raised systolic pressure about 16 percent and diastolic pressure 9 percent. Further, taking 1,000 milligrams of vitamin C a day has significantly reduced blood pressure.

Eating fruits and vegetables, especially fruit—full of vitamin C—also causes blood pressure to drop. Vegetarians generally have lower blood pressure than meat eaters. Indeed, eating a vegetarian diet for more than five years clearly helped overcome a genetic predisposition to high blood pressure in older African-Americans, according to research at Colorado State University.

WATCH THE SALTY STUFF

Here's another reason your blood pressure may go up as you age. Sodium. Sodium affects your blood pressure more as you get older, because nearly everyone becomes more sensitive to salt with age, and depending on genetic susceptibility, this could drive up your blood pressure, according to M. H. Weinberger, at the Hypertension Research Center at the Indiana University School of Medicine. In a ten-year study, he found a progressive increase in salt sensitivity in the entire population, although it came earlier in life and more dramatically to those who subsequently developed high blood pressure. In ordinary Americans, salt sensitivity did not increase until around age sixty. Salt sensitivity, then, is a function of age, but this does not mean high blood pressure need follow. Going easy on salt throughout life can stop the blood pressure–boosting effect of increased sodium sensitivity from kicking in. Also, other dietary factors, such as adequate calcium and potassium, can make you less salt sensitive.

HOW TO KEEP BLOOD PRESSURE DOWN AS YOU AGE

- ▲ Eat lots of fruits and vegetables. Fruit fiber is particularly potent, according to a four-year Harvard study of middle-aged and elderly men. Skimpy fruit eaters were 46 percent more apt to develop high blood pressure as they got older than men who ate the fiber found in five apples a day.
- ▲ Take supplements of vitamin C as insurance. Even 250 milligrams a day cuts your risk of high blood pressure as you age nearly in half, Tufts studies found.

▲ Don't get addicted to salt. For example, don't add salt to infant foods. Restrict processed foods; they contribute about 70 percent of sodium to typical diets. Eliminating one teaspoon of salt a day can reduce systolic pressure on average 7 mmHg and diastolic 3.5 mmHg in some people with high blood pressure.

▲ Eat red grapes and red or purple grape juice. Research at the University of Florida finds that grape chemicals help dilate arteries, and thus may reduce blood pressure.

▲ Eat a couple of stalks of celery a day. Chemicals in that amount of celery lowered blood pressure in animals, according to University of Chicago researchers. Celery is an ancient blood pressure treatment among traditional Vietnamese doctors.

▲ Eat garlic and/or take garlic pills. In a double-blind test, 600 milligrams of the German garlic preparation Kwai pushed blood pressure down from an average 171/102 to 152/89 within three months.

▲ Get lots of potassium. Without enough, you retain sodium, triggering high blood pressure. Temple University investigators found that blood pressure in potassium-restricted men jumped about 4.5 percent, up from 90.9 to 95 arterial pressure (a measure of both systolic and diastolic). Potassium is concentrated in fruits and vegetables, nuts, soybeans and fish.

▲ Eat oatmeal. Eating only one small bowl of oatmeal (about an ounce) a day lowered blood pressure, according to a study by Johns Hopkins University researchers. And the more oatmeal, the lower the blood pressure sank, regardless of age, weight, alcohol consumption and sodium or potassium intake. Probable agent: soluble fiber.

▲ Eat more fatty fish, such as salmon, mackerel and sardines, or take fish oil supplements under the supervision of a physician. In one University of Cincinnati test, blood pressure dropped 4.4 points diastolic and 6.5 points systolic in people taking 2,000 milligrams of omega-3 fatty acid in capsules for three months. That's about seven capsules a day. Each capsule typically contains 300 milligrams of actual fish oil—EPA and DHA.

▲ Get lots of calcium. The mineral helps block high blood pressure from salt sensitivity. In a test at the University of Texas Health Science Center, 800 milligrams of daily calcium depressed mild high blood pressure by 20 to 30 points in 20 percent of subjects.

▲ Get adequate magnesium. In a recent Dutch study, taking 485 milligrams of magnesium (aspartate) a day lowered blood pressure an average 2.7 mgmHg systolic and 3.4 diastolic in women with borderline to moderate high blood pressure.

▲ Restrict alcohol. It's one of the biggest unsuspected causes of high blood pressure, although the mechanism is unclear. Keep to under two drinks a day.

▲ If you are overweight, losing some pounds can be a fast treatment. One reason: Free radical activity picks up with too much fat consumption. Restricting calories turns down free radical production. Also, salt sensitivity is more common in the obese.

Note: Reducing sodium is not a universal cure-all. Cutting down on sodium and upping calcium can cause no change in blood pressure or, oddly, even cause it to rise in some individuals. Be sure to take your blood pressure regularly to ascertain that dietary changes have the desired effect.

———

*Three or more alcoholic drinks a day is the most
common cause of reversible or curable hypertension.*
—N. M. Kaplan, University of Texas Health Science
Center, Dallas

———

Who Says You
Have to Get Cataracts?

▲　▲　▲

Everybody knows cataracts are a phenomenon of getting old. Right? The figures show it: Only about 4.5 percent of Americans have cataracts in their fifties. By ages seventy and eighty, that figure has multiplied ten times—almost 50 percent have vision dimmed by cataracts. But is age the real culprit? And are cataracts really a necessary part of aging? Bluntly, such senile cataracts, like so many other infirmities as we get older, appear to stem from a vitamin deficiency, says Dr. Irwin H. Rosenberg, director of the USDA's Human Nutrition Research Center on Aging at Tufts. Or, more specifically, an antioxidant deficiency.

Yes, it's those destructive oxygen free radicals at work again. This time they have targeted the lens of the eyes. They are born of photooxidation that comes with simple exposure to ultraviolet light—or being in sunlight so the light strikes the lens of the eyes. It's normal, but after years, it takes a toll by oxidizing proteins, damaging crystalline in the lens, turning it opaque. That is, unless you have a plentiful supply of antioxidants in the lens to splice out the damaged crystalline so it does not build up into a cloudy lens.

It's rather clear-cut, says Dr. Rosenberg. A number of studies indicate that cataracts tend to come to people who get the least antioxidant vitamins and spare those who get the most. In particular, vitamin C seems most powerful in warding off cataracts. In one study he cites, Americans in the lowest one-third of vitamin C intake were fourteen times more apt to develop cataracts than those in the top third. Those getting the least vitamin E had a three times greater rate of cataracts; those skimping on beta carotene had a one and a half times greater risk for cataracts as they aged.

In other recent research at the State University of New York at Stony Brook, investigators found that relatively high intakes of antioxidant nutrients corresponded with low risk of cataracts in a group of nearly 1,400 people, ages forty to seventy. Also, those who took multivitamin supplements at least once a week for at least a year were less apt to develop cataracts as they aged than non–vitamin takers.

Nor do you have to suffer macular degeneration, a serious degeneration of the eye's macula, leading to blindness. A recent study by Michael S. Kaminski at the Pacific University College of Optometry in Oregon reported that 92 percent of a group of men and women with macular degeneration were deficient in at least one antioxidant nutrient. Seventy-five percent lacked two or more, most notably vitamin E, zinc and selenium. Research shows that nearly everybody over age fifty-five lacks at least one of the major antioxidants thought to protect against macular degeneration, and three-quarters are deficient in all three.

A study at the National Eye Institute showed that people with the highest blood levels of fruit and vegetable chemicals called carotenoids, including beta carotene, were only one-third as apt to develop macular degeneration as those with the lowest carotenoid levels. Even those who ate moderate amounts of carotenoids cut their odds of macular degeneration in half. A carotenoid called lutein may be particularly powerful, according to Swiss researchers. They have found lutein highly concentrated in the macula, the part of the eye responsible for sharp vision. They theorize that antioxidant lutein and other carotenoids fight off oxygen free radicals that can damage the macula, destroying sight. Interestingly, vegetables highest in lutein are kale, spinach and collard greens.

In animal studies, vitamin C, vitamin E and beta carotene have been especially protective against macular degeneration.

How to Keep Your Vision as You Age

Take Multivitamins: Just taking a one-a-day vitamin-mineral supplement could cut your chances of having cataracts 27 percent. That was the surprise finding from a study of about eighteen thousand male physicians by Harvard researchers who tracked the men over a ten-year period. Another study at the University of Melbourne in Australia found that the progression of cataracts was slowed in men with long-term histories of vitamin supplement use.

Take Vitamin C: In a Canadian study, those who took vitamin C and vitamin E supplements were less apt to develop cataracts. How much? Probably 500 milligrams a day of vitamin C is optimum to keep cataracts away, and you don't get added protection by taking more, say Tufts researchers. Nobody is sure of the best doses of vitamin E and beta carotene to combat cataracts.

Eat Greens: A recent study in the *British Medical Journal* found spinach the one food most closely linked to preventing cataracts in a large group of older women. Beta carotene, high in spinach, may be one reason. Women in the study who ate the most beta carotene foods were only

40 percent as apt to develop cataracts. The study also heralded vitamin C supplements as preventing cataracts.
Women who took 250 to 500 milligrams of vitamin C daily
for ten years were about half as likely to have cataracts as
non–vitamin takers.

Your Ultimate Plan
for Slowing Down
and Reversing Aging

▲   ▲   ▲   ▲   ▲   ▲   ▲

It would be easy if you could just take one antiaging pill and be done with it. But there's no such thing. No single vitamin, mineral, herb, food or other substance known to science has everything you need to ward off aging. The more they investigate, the more scientists understand that nature works with a subtle synergy in which elements support and potentiate each other to achieve the most powerful impact on cell functioning. The Lone Ranger attack, the single silver-bullet cure that we expect from pharmaceutical drugs, is not the best in complex matters of fighting aging and prolonging life.

There's no magic bullet. It's not just one [vitamin] or another; they're all important. —Dr. Gladys Block, University of California at Berkeley

It's an illusion to imagine a single all-purpose antioxidant. —Dr. Jerome DeCosse, Memorial Sloan-Kettering Cancer Center, New York

You must raise levels of many antioxidants to best deter aging, because they all work together to protect cells against free radical damage and other contributors to premature aging. What's really important is your overall antioxidant status. Do you have enough of the right type of antioxidants to optimally defend your cells against free radical assaults at any instant? Obviously, there are no complete answers in this frontier-era of scientific investigation into aging. Nobody knows how much we will eventually be able to do to conquer aging. Thus, it's impossible to get full protection against premature aging. But you can certainly give yourself the most basic insurance against needless aging, based on the best current knowledge.

Antiaging Supplement Strategy

▲ ▲ ▲

Here, according to the latest scientific evidence, are the ten best supplements you can take to delay or reverse many of the common signs of needless aging.

1. MULTIVITAMIN PILL: Take a standard multivitamin-mineral pill that provides about 100 percent of the RDA (recommended dietary allowance) for most of the vitamins, minerals and trace elements. This supplement alone can do wonders for many people, correcting unsuspected deficiencies, particularly boosting immunity to infections that are often devastating in older people. If you take no other supplements, take this one.

Note: Look for a multi with at least 100 percent of the RDA for B vitamins, including 400 micrograms of folic acid. Also try to find a multi with no more than 100 percent of the RDA for iron, and less if possible, if you are a postmenopausal woman or a man. Excess iron can promote aging. Under a new labeling law, effective December 1996, the term "daily value," or DV, will be used instead of RDA on supplement labels. You may see DV on the labels of some brands before that time.

2. VITAMIN E: This is an essential antioxidant vitamin because there is virtually no way you can get enough vitamin E in food to protect cells against free radical damage and ward off heart disease, cancer, declining immunity and other chronic diseases of aging, including possibly brain degeneration. Vitamin E is a nonspecific antioxidant that generally guards cells from oxidative damage. Most standard multi pills contain no more than 30 units of E— not nearly enough to save you from premature aging. Unless you find high antiaging doses in a multi supplement, you need separate vitamin E pills to get a daily dose of 100 to 400 IU.

3. VITAMIN C: Vitamin C is one of the antioxidant staples required by your cells to retard many conditions of aging. People who get the most vitamin C, some in supplements, have been shown to have slightly longer life spans. Most experts recommend doses of at least 500 to 1,000 milligrams of vitamin C daily—and more if you want. This almost always requires a separate pill. Standard multi pills contain only 60 milligrams of C.

4. BETA CAROTENE: Beta carotene is one of the triumvirate of antioxidant staples, along with vitamin E and vitamin C. The three work together synergistically to maintain high antioxidant activity in cells. You can get very high doses of beta carotene in dark orange vegetables and fruits and dark leafy green vegetables. For some people this can be sufficient. However, many antioxidant researchers take a beta carotene supplement of 10 to 15 milligrams daily as antiaging insurance.

Caution: Be sure to get pills labeled beta carotene and not plain vitamin A. Few multi tablets have high doses of beta carotene. You will probably need a separate tablet.

5. CHROMIUM: This mineral supplement is essential because it is virtually impossible to get enough chromium in food to ward off detrimental aging changes. It is usually left out of multi pills or included only in very low amounts. You will probably need a separate chromium pill. Recommended dose: 200 micrograms daily.

6. SELENIUM: Selenium is regarded as a potential anti-cancer agent, heart protector and, most recently, a suppressor of viruses, including the AIDS virus. Selenium is usually not put into multivitamin-mineral pills in adequate doses, so you will probably need a separate pill. Suggested antiaging doses: 50 to 200 micrograms daily.

Caution: Selenium in high doses is toxic.

7. CALCIUM: Unless you eat or drink lots of dairy products, it is difficult to get enough calcium to ward off the troubles of aging. Recommended daily dose for most adults: at least 1,000 milligrams. Postmenopausal women need 1,500 milligrams along with 200 to 600 IU of vitamin D. A separate calcium supplement is needed. You cannot get enough calcium in multi tablets.

8. ZINC: This mineral is critical for proper immune functioning as you age and can reverse failing immunity due to aging changes. Recommended doses: 15 to 30 milligrams daily. Many multivitamins contain 15 milligrams. High doses of zinc can suppress immune functions and can have other detrimental effects.

9. MAGNESIUM: Most Americans appear deficient in magnesium, which may help prevent heart disease—especially arrhythmias and congestive heart failure. In animals, magnesium also helps prevent free radical damage to cells. You usually get about 25 percent of the recommended daily amounts in multi tablets. You may want to take a separate magnesium tablet of 200 to 300 milligrams daily if you don't eat a high-magnesium diet.

10. COENZYME Q-10: This is a general antioxidant,

TEN BASIC PILLS TO KEEP YOU YOUNG

Here's what most healthy adults need daily to stop aging now, according to the latest research:

- ▲ Multivitamin-mineral tablet with about 100 percent of the RDA for most vitamins, minerals and trace elements.
- ▲ Vitamin E (100 to 400 IU)
- ▲ Vitamin C (500 to 1,500 milligrams)
- ▲ Beta carotene (10 to 15 milligrams)
- ▲ Chromium (200 micrograms)
- ▲ Calcium (500 to 1,500 milligrams)
- ▲ Zinc (15 to 30 milligrams)*
- ▲ Selenium (50 to 200 micrograms)
- ▲ Magnesium (200 to 300 milligrams)
- ▲ Coenzyme Q-10 (30 milligrams)

Note: You can usually get enough antiaging B vitamins, including folic acid, in a multivitamin-mineral pill. However, you may need separate B vitamin tablets in higher doses for specific health reasons. (For more details, see pages 68–80.)

Important: The doses given are in ranges and how much you take depends on your individual circumstances. Do not fall into the trap that more is always better. In some cases, high doses can be toxic and detrimental. Be sure to check with a physician before taking high doses of individual supplements if you are on medications, are pregnant or have any kind of health problem. Supplements can interact with medications to produce adverse effects.

* 15 milligrams of zinc are often found in multivitamin-mineral supplements.

somewhat like vitamin E, and is now being acclaimed by researchers on antioxidants. It preserves youth in laboratory animals. It is thought to have particular energy-stimulating effects on heart muscle cells and has long been used in Europe and Japan to treat heart failure. It comes in various types of tablets and capsules. Standard anti-aging dose: 30 milligrams daily, more if you have heart failure or other cardiovascular problems (see page 138).

OTHER ANTIAGING SUPPLEMENTS TO CONSIDER IF YOU ARE MIDDLE-AGED (FORTY TO FIFTY) OR OLDER OR HAVE SYMPTOMS OF SPECIFIC AGE-RELATED DISEASES

B VITAMINS: These are far more critical than previously suspected as guardians against mental deterioration, heart disease and cancer. You can get fairly good antiaging doses in multivitamin pills, which may be enough for the general population. However, to be on the safe side, especially if you are past forty or have specific health worries related to a lack of B vitamins, you may need higher doses, which are available only in individual pills. This includes 500 to 1,000 micrograms of vitamin B12, 1,000 micrograms of folic acid and up to 50 milligrams of vitamin B6.

GINKGO: This herb supplement should be taken as needed to improve blood circulation to all vessels, including those in the brain, heart and limbs. A standard dose for those with declining functions due to aging: a 40-milligram tablet three times a day.

GLUTATHIONE: Taking antioxidant glutathione is good insurance to keep oxidized fats in foods from getting through your gastrointestinal tract and into circulation in your body. Glutathione fortifies cells in the GI tract, providing a barrier against the free-radical-producing fats. A 100-milligram tablet of glutathione daily should be protective. Be sure to take it with meals.

GLUTAMINE: Glutamine is an amino acid that should be taken in high doses as needed at times of stress or illness, or if you have a specific reason, such as muscle weakness and deterioration. Some experts take an antiaging dose of 2,000 to 8,000 milligrams daily.

FISH OIL CONCENTRATE IN CAPSULES: If you do not eat fish, a daily dose of 1,000 milligrams of a combination of DHA and EPA fatty acids, as noted on the label, equals the amount of omega-3 fatty acids in about three and a half ounces of salmon, sardines or mackerel. Be sure also to take vitamin E. Don't take fish oil capsules without consulting a physician if you have any type of clotting or bleeding problems or are on anticoagulant medications.

GARLIC SUPPLEMENTS: If you don't eat garlic, or even if you do, take three to six capsules of garlic powder or extract a day as a general antiaging dose.

L-CARNITINE: If you have angina, heart arrhythmias or mild signs of heart failure, you may want to take l-carnitine, an amino acid, under a doctor's supervision. Doses of 1,000 to 2,000 milligrams daily have been used to combat congestive heart failure.

Antiaging Diet Strategy

▲ ▲ ▲

Here's what to eat and not eat to give yourself the best chances of arriving at an old age in good shape:

1. EAT FRUITS AND VEGETABLES: Of all things you can do to retard aging, this is number one because it gives you the greatest amounts and range of antioxidants. Eat as many fruits and vegetables as you can of a great variety— at least five servings a day. These infuse your blood with a steady stream of free radical–fighting antioxidants, some known, many yet to be discovered. If you start young—in childhood—you blunt many of the early physiological changes (such as clogged arteries) and cellular damage that accumulate as premature aging. By midlife, the antioxidant protection of fruits and vegetables is critical to keep you from sliding into degenerative diseases of aging. Even at a late age, fruits and vegetables still give your cells ammunition to halt the progression of damage that brings on disease and early death.

2. EAT FISH: You should eat fish at least twice or three times a week. Any fish is beneficial, but the fatty fish, salmon, mackerel, sardines, tuna and herring, have the most antiaging omega-3 type fatty acids.

3. DRINK TEA: Of all beverages, tea is the most acclaimed as an antiaging beverage. It's full of antioxidants.

4. EAT SOYBEAN FOODS: If eating soybean foods once a day is not possible, eat them at least two or three times a week. The soybean contains many antioxidants and other substances particularly thought to deter certain cancers.

5. RESTRICT CALORIES: Eat only enough calories for proper growth and optimum nutrition. If you can restrict calories after adulthood and maintain a lower than "normal" weight, your chances of retaining your youth and living longer go up dramatically. Do not restrict calories to below-normal amounts in growing children or elderly or ill adults who need nutrients from more calories.

6. RESTRICT THE WRONG FATS: Avoid cell-damaging fats, such as meat and dairy fat, and in particular polyunsaturated fats and partially hydrogenated fats in margarines, many vegetable oils and processed foods. Use almost exclusively olive oil, canola oil and other monounsaturated oils, such as macadamia nut oil.

7. GO EASY ON MEAT: Restrict or avoid meat and cook it in ways to avoid the creation of free radicals as much as possible (see pages 219–225).

8. CONSIDER THE PROS AND CONS OF ALCOHOL: Do not drink excessive amounts of alcohol, which is a free radical factory. If you do drink moderately, make it primarily wine, especially red wine containing various antioxidants from grapes—no more than one or two glasses a day.

9. CURB SWEETS: Do not eat excessive amounts of sugar or other carbohydrates, including fructose, which raises blood insulin levels, damaging arteries and possibly promoting cancer, as well as other degenerative diseases.

10. EAT GARLIC: It's one of the most ancient, respected carriers of various antioxidants. Remarkable studies in animals and humans suggest it inhibits cancer, artery clogging and perhaps degenerative brain function due to aging. A clove a day, raw or cooked, is an appropriate anti-aging dose.

QUESTIONS

Who's Deficient? Anybody who is needlessly vulnerable to premature aging and suffering or death from chronic diseases that could be prevented, postponed or reversed by taking and eating more of specific natural chemicals. That is virtually everybody in our modern society, since we are all aging much more rapidly than is decreed by the passage of time.

When Should You Start Antiaging Supplements? Now, if you are age eighteen or older—no matter how much older you are. As Dr. Denham Harman, free radical authority at the University of Nebraska, says, "Aging starts at conception," and you have at least seven, eight or even nine decades in which to intervene to prevent or reverse the cellular damage that leads to premature and needless aging. Sure, it's better to start taking antiaging supplements early in life. Some studies show that taking certain supplements for fifteen years offers more protection than taking them for one year. But it's better to start sometime than never. Vitamins and minerals have revived immunity in the very elderly, reversed "senility" and prevented many broken bones and irreversible disability even in people over age eighty.

"I think it makes sense to pay special attention to your diet, increasing intake of nutritional foods, *before you reach old age,*" says Tufts antioxidant authority Dr. Jeffrey Blumberg. His theory is that if you can retard or reverse a phenomenon like the decline in immunity with nutritional intervention in older adults, it's reasonable to speculate we can slow age-related changes by having a relatively high intake of these nutrients in middle years.

What About Children? As insurance against vitamin-mineral deficiencies and a poor diet, children can take a one-a-day vitamin-mineral pill. Some experts believe that "priming" children with antioxidants at an early age may help save them from premature aging and aging diseases later in life. It makes sense, according to the free radical theory of aging and animal experiments. However, since virtually no studies have been done on the effects of antioxidants on growing children, most experts shy away from sanctioning such high doses of supplements for youngsters. Nevertheless, studies show that many children lack common vitamins, which makes them susceptible to childhood infections and other diseases. A one-a-day tablet, containing about 100 percent of the RDA for vitamins and minerals, can prevent such deficiencies.

Two reasonable exceptions:

▲ Aging bones: Recent research finds that the time to intervene to guarantee strong bones later in life is right before or during puberty. Thus calcium supplements for young girls especially may protect against disintegration of bone in old age.

▲ Breast cancer: Surprisingly, it appears that the stage may be set for breast cancer in a woman's early years—between ages fourteen and twenty-five. Evidence suggests that an anticancer diet of lots of fruits and vegetables and antioxidants in late adolescence and early adulthood may be particularly critical in warding off breast cancer later in life.

What About Pregnant Women? Certainly, taking vitamins, in particular folic acid, in the early days of pregnancy—

even before you know you are pregnant—can prevent birth defects, such as spina bifida, an incomplete fusion of the brain and spinal cord. Thus, all women of child-bearing ages should take at least 400 micrograms of folic acid, available in a multivitamin-mineral pill.

However, what supplements to take *during* pregnancy is a matter of some concern among scientists. Most obstetrician-gynecologists do recommend a prenatal multivitamin-mineral supplement during pregnancy. It's known that high doses of retinol-type vitamin A (not beta carotene) can be detrimental during pregnancy and should be avoided. As for antioxidant supplements, such as beta carotene, vitamin C and vitamin E, Dr. Jeffrey Blumberg, antioxidant authority at Tufts, says daily doses of up to 400 IU of vitamin E, 1,000 milligrams of vitamin C and up to 15 milligrams of beta carotene should be as beneficial to pregnant women as other women and pose no hazard. Theoretically, exposure to antioxidants in the womb should also be beneficial to the fetus if animal studies hold up. In animal experiments, such offspring tend to live longer.

Nevertheless, since data on the effects on the human fetus are lacking, it's unknown what doses of antioxidants as well as other antiaging supplements may be beneficial or harmful, says leading free radical expert Dr. Denham Harman. He advises pregnant women to eat a diet high in antioxidant-rich fruits and vegetables, but to be cautious and *not* take megadoses of various antiaging vitamins, minerals, nutrients, herbs and other supplements except on the advice of a physician.

All pregnant women should consult their physicians about which supplements to use and in what amounts.

What If You Are on Medications? Don't stop taking conventional medications and/or substitute antioxidants or other supplements to treat a specific health condition, except on the advice of your doctor. In some cases, taking certain supplements may ultimately enable a person to take lower doses of medications or even drop them entirely, but this decision should be made only after consultation with your physician or other professional health adviser. There also can be interactions between supplements and specific medications, so if you are on any medications, check with a physician before adding supplements.

Do Supplements Contain What They Say? There have been many horror stories suggesting that vitamins, since they are not regulated as drugs by the Food and Drug Administration, are substandard, do not contain the active ingredients claimed on the label and don't dissolve properly in your body. However, Consumers Union, as reported in their September 1994 issue of *Consumer Reports*, tested eighty-six nutritional supplements—both multivitamin-mineral formulas and single-ingredient supplements—and discovered that virtually all passed their tests. Consumers Union used the standards of the U.S. Pharmacopoeia (USP), an independent organization that sets voluntary standards for vitamin and mineral manufacture.

"With one exception, all of the multivitamin-mineral and single supplement products we tested generally contained the amounts stated on their labels and disintegrated within an acceptable time period," concluded *Consumer Reports*.

They also said that cheaper vitamins and mineral supplements are just as effective as expensive ones. Their survey found that the American Association of Retired Persons' (AARP) 101 Hi-Potency supplement was the most inexpensive entry and cost about one-fifth as much as the most expensive one—Shaklee. But both brands had comparable ingredients.

Other tips: Look for an expiration date on your supplements, and don't use them past that date. Store in a cool dry place, such as a kitchen cupboard. Take multiple supplements with meals, not on an empty stomach, to get optimal absorption. You need a little fat to get the best utilization of fat-soluble beta carotene or vitamin A, vitamin E and vitamin D. Some multiple tablets come in divided doses, which are excellent because they infuse your blood with steady supplies of vitamins all day long.

Last Word: Obviously there are no final and complete answers on postponing aging at this point. Nobody at this early stage knows how far we can push the envelope when it comes to preserving and retrieving youth and vitality. As for the optimum antiaging doses of supplements, scientists simply can't be exact but can suggest only a range of doses, based on the best current but incomplete research. Since this is the first time humankind has attempted to slow down the aging process by diet and supplements, the first suggestions are apt to be modest so as not to be unduly hazardous. They may turn out to be too conservative.

But they offer science's most exciting prospects to help you stop aging now! It's a gamble that could pay off as no other can—with a longer life, less suffering, disease and disability, and more happiness and joy at being alive.

More Reasons Why You Can Stop Aging Now!

▲   ▲   ▲   ▲   ▲   ▲   ▲

Since *Stop Aging Now!* was first published in August 1995, new research has continued to confirm the powerful antiaging activity in antioxidant foods and supplements, as well as cautions to current smokers about taking very high doses of beta carotene.

Here are some of the highlights.

NEW CREDIBILITY FOR VITAMIN E

There's exciting new proof that high doses of vitamin E, as recommended in this book, can thwart heart attacks to an astonishing extent. In a landmark study, researchers at Cambridge University in England showed for the first time that taking daily doses of 400 IU or 800 IU slashed non-fatal heart attacks by a startling 77 percent. In fact, vitamin E was more powerful in warding off such heart attacks than cholesterol-lowering drugs and aspirin, said researchers Professor Morris Brown and Dr. Malcolm Michinson. In their double-blind study of 2,000 patients with confirmed coronary artery disease, half of the group got vitamin E and half got a placebo (dummy pill) for an average eighteen months.

The result: those taking vitamin E suffered only 23 percent as many non-fatal heart attacks as those not taking vitamin E. Indeed, researchers found vitamin E-takers no more vulnerable to such heart attacks than healthy individuals with no signs of heart disease. In other words, vitamin E turned back the clock of many heart disease patients to pre-heart disease days—and in the incredibly short time of a year and a half or less! Benefits were evident as early as six and a half months after starting vitamin E, researchers reported. However, vitamin E did not reduce cardiovascular deaths, possibly because the vitamin is less effective against the frequent cause of such deaths (arrhythmias and progressive heart failure); vitamin E primarily fights formation of arterial plaque and clots. Note: the vitamin E used in the study was the natural form, not synthetic. It was taken in a single daily dose.

In another new study at the University of Bern in Switzerland, researchers have discovered a new way vitamin E discourages artery clogging. It's well known that vitamin E helps block toxic changes (oxidation) that enable bad-type LDL cholesterol to clog arteries. But the vitamin also helps keep arteries open by inhibiting the proliferation of smooth muscle cells that contributes to clogged arteries. The Swiss researchers demonstrated that rabbits given vitamin E had only half as much damage to the aortas of their hearts as rabbits not given vitamin E. Indeed, vitamin E both prevented the occurrence of so-called fatty streaks, the earliest sign of artery damage— and kept artery damage from progressing once it occurred later in life. Thus, it's clear that plenty of vitamin E, which you can only get from supplements, is needed both early and throughout life to keep arteries open and flexible.

New Beta Carotene Puzzles

New evidence supports the caution (page 65) that ultra-high doses of beta carotene supplements may, for unknown reasons, encourage lung cancer in smokers. A recent study at the University of Washington in Seattle (the so-called CARET study) found that high amounts of synthetic beta carotene—50 milligrams a day—plus 25,000 IU of vitamin A daily boosted the risk of lung cancer in smokers and those exposed to asbestos by 42 percent. However, those who quit smoking before the study began and then took beta carotene supplements actually showed a 20 percent lower risk of lung cancer.

More researchers now warn current smokers against taking single high doses of beta carotene supplements until the reasons for the seemingly detrimental effects of beta carotene are clarified. The Council for Responsible Nutrition advises smokers to stick with the low doses of beta carotene found in food and in most multivitamin-mineral tablets—3 to 6 milligrams a day.

At the same time, preliminary results of the large-scale Harvard physicians study did not find that taking 50 milligrams of synthetic beta carotene every other day prevented cancer or heart attacks. Study chief Charles Hennekens said he was disappointed in the finding, but did not advise people who are taking beta carotene supplements to stop taking them. Dr. Jeffrey Blumberg, antioxidant authority at Tufts University, emphasizes that about two hundred other studies do demonstrate benefits from beta carotene; he continues to take 15 milligrams of beta carotene daily. The Alliance for Aging Research says

10 milligrams may be enough, although it sees no hazards for nonsmoking adults in the higher doses it has previously suggested (page 61). What the new research confirms, says Dr. Blumberg, is that neither beta carotene nor any other single antioxidant is a "magic bullet"; you need many antioxidants working together to protect and detoxify cells. Thus, new research reinforces the wisdom of eating a high-antioxidant diet, including foods high in beta carotene, and taking a variety of supplemental antioxidants, including vitamin E and vitamin C, as outlined in this book.

In another ongoing study, Harvard researcher JoAnn Manson, M.D. is giving supplements of beta carotene, vitamin E and vitamin C to 8,000 women at high risk of heart disease. She has seen no evidence of harm to the women from beta carotene and says there is good reason to believe beta carotene (as well as the other antioxidants) "may benefit them." She notes that beta carotene, in addition to acting as an antioxidant, appears to relax artery walls, helping keep arteries flexible and less clogged.

Alarming New B Vitamin Deficiencies

Startling new evidence shows that vitamin B deficiencies in older people are far worse than previously suspected. This can lead to memory loss, depression, and pseudo symptoms of Alzheimer's disease, as well as heart attacks and strokes (page 68). A new study of three hundred subjects between sixty-five and ninety-six years old revealed "epidemic" vitamin B deficiencies, according to researchers at six medical centers around the world, including Columbia Presbyterian Medical Center in New York. The deficiencies were detected by special tests; unfortunately, standard blood tests proclaimed B vitamin levels "normal."

The hidden deficiencies had serious consequences; for example, an astonishing 92 percent of the subjects had B vitamin deficiencies, leading to abnormally high levels of homocysteine, a blood protein increasingly incriminated in heart disease and strokes. Daily injections of 1 milligram of B12, 1.1 milligrams of folic acid, and 5 milligrams of B6 eliminated the hazard in only five to twelve days! Oral supplements are also expected to correct the problem.

Most important in controlling homocysteine is folic acid. Upping intake of folic acid could prevent up to fifty thousand deaths from heart disease every year, according to a new analysis of thirty-eight studies by Shirley Beresford, University of Washington.

Message: Ordinary blood tests don't reveal B deficiencies, and people past middle age must take supplements to get adequate doses of B vitamins to ward off the awful consequences of potential B deficiencies that worsen with age.

NEW ZINC POWERS REVEALED

Zinc, hailed for its powers to boost immune functioning, notably in older people, by revitalizing the thymus gland (page 92), is far more essential in combating free radicals and general overall aging than previously known, according to new studies by Debasis Bagchi of Creighton University School of Pharmacy and Allied Health. Dr. Bagchi tested several forms of the mineral—zinc gluconate, zinc picolinate, zinc sulfate, zinc citrate, zinc oxide, and zinc methionine. He found that zinc methionine (sold as OptiZinc) was up to ten times more effective than other zinc forms in neutralizing free radicals. Indeed, zinc methionine equaled powerful vitamin E and vitamin C in antioxidant strength. Least effective were zinc oxide and zinc citrate. That means the right type of zinc can help ward off overall bodily disintegration. Check the label of supplements for the type of zinc used.

Magnesium Strengthens Heart, Calms Brain

Evidence pours in that too little magnesium makes you more susceptible to heart disease and diabetes. A new study of fifteen thousand men and women, ages forty-five to sixty-four, by University of Minnesota researchers found that those with existing cardiovascular disease, high blood pressure, and diabetes had significantly lower blood levels of magnesium than those free of such diseases. Women with low blood levels of magnesium were more apt to have high bad-type LDL cholesterol and thickening of the walls of the carotid arteries, indicating arteries are clogged. Those with high dietary and blood magnesium had higher good-type HDL cholesterol as well as lower levels of blood sugar and insulin, a hormone that damages artery walls.

Your brain also needs magnesium to function well, according to new tests by research psychologist James G. Penland, at the U.S. Department of Agriculture. Even marginal deficiencies can overexcite brain cells, disturbing brain activity, as shown by electroencephalograms (EEG). For six months one group of women consumed only 115 milligrams of magnesium daily, or about 40 percent of the RDA for the mineral. After only six weeks, EEG readings showed overexcitability in brain cells of those low in magnesium. Researchers note that magnesium is abundant in the brain and is essential in regulating central nervous system excitability. They point out that people severely deficient in magnesium report epilepsy-type convulsions, dizziness, and muscle tremors as well as psychological symptoms, such as irritability, anxiety, confusion, depression, apathy, and insomnia.

Selenium Boosts Mood and Energy

Getting more of the trace mineral selenium may lift your mood and make you feel more energetic, Agriculture's Dr. Penland has also found. Men who boosted selenium intake in the diet to 220 micrograms a day had improved moods, even though they were not "deficient" in selenium to begin with, he reported. Dr. Penland also noted that the more selenium in the men's red blood cells—as determined by increased activity in a selenium-containing enzyme—the better they felt. The men with the more active enzymes felt more agreeable, less confused, less anxious, more confident and more energetic. Men with the lowest moods to begin with got the biggest benefits from the increased selenium.

Although the increase in mood-boosting selenium came from food, Dr. Penland says supplements would have the same effect. Obviously, many Americans lack the optimal selenium needed for peak well-being, he concluded.

Ginkgo Reverses Impotence

Ginkgo biloba, the herb that helps restore memory and prevent mental decline (page 148), may also combat another distressing problem that often afflicts aging men: sexual impotence. The reason: Ginkgo not only dilates blood vessels in the brain and extremities, it also improves blood flow to the penis, required for erections.

A recent study by German urologists found that 78 percent of fifty men suffering from "arterial erectile impotence" improved after taking 240 milligrams of ginkgo biloba extract daily for nine months. Blood flow to penile arteries generally improved after three months. Twenty men regained spontaneous erections after six months. Nineteen men regained potency when ginkgo was given with certain drug injections. Eleven remained impotent. In a previous study, the researchers reported some improvement from lower daily doses of 60 milligrams of ginkgo. There were no side effects from either dose, said researchers at the University Clinics of RWTH in Aachen.

GARLIC SHRINKS TUMORS

Garlic's powers may be stronger than expected in fighting existing cancer as well as in preventing its occurrence. Specific garlic chemicals have actually helped shut down the growth of tumors grown from human colon cancer cells. In new tests, scientists at Pennsylvania State University first transplanted human colon-cancer cells in mice. Then they treated some of the mice with a corn oil solution containing diallyl disulfide, or DADS, a chemical found in processed garlic. Other mice got plain corn oil. Remarkably, the tumors in mice getting the garlic chemical shrank by 60 percent. The tumors in mice given only corn oil continued to grow steadily. Previous Penn State research has shown that the garlic sulfur compound destroyed human colon, lung and skin tumor cells grown in lab cultures.

NEW ACCLAIM FOR TOMATOES

The fame of the antioxidant lycopene, found primarily in tomatoes, continues to grow. New tests by British researchers found lycopene four times stronger than other vegetable antioxidants in neutralizing the cell-damaging, cancer-promoting effects of cigarette smoke. Hawaiian investigators showed that lycopene actually destroyed cancer cells in test-tube experiments.

A new study by Harvard's Edward Giovannucci published in the Journal of the National Cancer Institute credited lycopene, the red color in tomatoes, with reducing the chances of prostate cancer. Among forty-eight thousand doctors and health professionals, those who ate at least ten servings of tomato-based foods a week were 35 percent less apt to get prostate cancer than those who ate less than one and one half servings a week. Most strongly linked to lower cancer risk was tomato sauce, followed by tomatoes and pizza.

New analyses by U.S. Department of Agriculture chemists have defined which tomato products have the most lycopene. Here are the milligrams of lycopene per serving of tomato products: one cup tomato soup (27 milligrams); one-half cup tomato sauce (22 milligrams); two tablespoons of tomato paste (21 milligrams); one-half cup tomato puree (21 milligrams); one-half cup spaghetti sauce (20 milligrams); three-quarters cup tomato juice (20 milligrams); one medium red ripe tomato (11 milligrams); one-half cup canned tomatoes (11 milligrams); two tablespoons ketchup (5 milligrams).

Also on the market now are lycopene supplements.

FISH'S MIGHTY ANTIAGING POWERS CONFIRMED

A new study at the University of Washington in Seattle finds that eating fish seems to do more than protect arteries from clogging; it also helps prevent deadly cardiac arrest—stoppage of the heart—caused by sudden fibrillation or irregular contractions of heart muscle. Such stoppage often comes without any previous warning of heart disease and kills about 250,000 Americans a year. In a study of more than eight hundred people, investigators found that those who ate small amounts of fatty fish, such as salmon, herring, and mackerel—even one serving a week—reduced their likelihood of cardiac arrest by a remarkable 50 to 70 percent!

At the same time, a recent twelve-year Harvard study noted that eating high amounts of fish did not seem to reduce heart disease in men any more than eating low amounts of fish. The implication is that even a little fish may provide potent protection, and that eating more fish (such as every day) has little or no added benefit.

Brain Protector: According to new exciting research, fish oil seems essential to protecting both developing and aging brains. One researcher noted that the brains of Alzheimer's patients had abnormally low levels of omega–3 fatty acids. "The old saying that fish is brain food is true," says researcher Norman Salem Jr., at the National Institute of Alcohol Abuse and Alcoholism. He concludes that DHA, one fatty acid component of fish oil (high in salmon), helps stave off depression, brain damage from alcohol, and other age-related brain diseases. For one reason: Studies show that DHA fish fat in brain-cell membranes helps regulate neurotransmitters, including critical serotonin, known to be lacking in those with depression and other neurological diseases.

Life Extender: When Dr. Gabriel Fernandes at the University of Texas Health Science Center in San Antonio fed lab mice omega–3 fatty acids found in fish, the mice lived from 33 percent to 50 percent longer than mice not getting the fish oil. Even more impressive was the possible explanation. Dr. Fernandes discovered that the fish omega–3 oils actually revved up production of three antiaging enzymes—catalase, superoxide dismutase, and glutathione peroxidase. Thus, fish oil appears to stimulate powerful internal defenses against youth-destroying free radicals.

Cancer Blocker: Eating a diet high in fish slowed the spread of human breast cancers injected into mice by more than 50 percent compared with corn oil, according to tests at the American Health Foundation. Also, tumors in fish-oil-fed mice were only two-thirds as large as those in corn-fed animals.

It's Always Teatime

Adding to the evidence that drinking tea fights aging by protecting the heart and arteries is a new study from Japan, reported in the British Medical Journal. Among 1,371 Japanese men over age forty, those who drank the most green tea had the lowest total blood cholesterol and triglycerides and best ratio of good HDL cholesterol to bad LDL cholesterol. Further, the amount of oxidized or dangerous-type fats in the blood dropped, the more tea the men drank. In fact, heavy smokers who drank more than ten small-size Japanese cups of green tea daily had no more oxidized blood fats than nonsmokers. This suggests the tea neutralized harmful free radicals that promote clogging. Moreover, green tea drinkers had less evidence of liver cell damage, including lower iron stores; higher iron promotes damage and accelerates aging.

Drinking green tea may also help explain why Asian men who smoke more cigarettes than American men nevertheless have lower lung cancer death rates. So speculates I. P. Lee and colleagues at the Food and Drug

Administration. They discovered that green tea drinkers in Korea generally have relatively lower rates of cancer-causing genetic damage to cells (cell mutations) despite the fact that they smoke. Remarkably, smokers who drank green tea had the same low frequency of mutations as nonsmokers, whereas smokers who did not drink tea or who drank coffee had high rates of cell mutations leading to cancer. This suggests that antioxidants in green tea may partially counteract smoke's harm to body cells.

When experts say tea fights aging, they mean real tea, not herbal teas, and there's new evidence why. Numerous tests show that regular tea—ordinary black and green teas found in any grocery store—is full of antioxidants. Herbal teas are not. In a recent analysis, British researchers at Trinity College in Dublin detected only one-tenth to one-fourth as much tannins (common antioxidants) in thirty-nine commercial herbal teas as in real teas. Only one herbal tea even came close: bearberry tea. Other tea herbs with the most tannins were mate, blackberry, and peppermint. Peppermint contained about one-fourth the antioxidant power of regular tea.

In the past, herbal teas were viewed as better for your health than regular teas, but science now says that's not true. Although herbal teas may have specific therapeutic benefits, regular tea is by far a better overall antiaging and health drink. Both caffeinated and decaffeinated teas have similar antioxidant activity.

SURPRISING NEW OLIVE BENEFITS

Eating olive oil instead of other fats protects not only your arteries but your cells against cancer, according to a new report in the Journal of the National Cancer Institute. Italian researchers found that using olive oil daily as a dressing on salads, vegetables and other foods cut the risk of lung cancer by 85 percent, as shown by an analysis of the diets of people with and without the disease. Interestingly, using olive oil in cooking did not protect against the cancer, possibly because heating olive oil destroys some of its antioxidants, researchers speculate.

And there's good news about olives per se. Surprisingly, olives contain high levels of unique polyphenolic antioxidants, similar to those in red wine and tea, according to new tests by Dr. Claudio Galli of the University of Milan. Dr. Galli calls the olive chemicals "very potent" in detoxifying dangerous LDL blood cholesterol that otherwise can lead to clogged arteries. Another plus for the arteries: The olive chemicals "at very low levels" help block platelet aggregation, a first step in clot formation that can trigger heart attacks and strokes. Aspirin has a similar effect in "thinning the blood."

Black olives contain much higher concentrations of the antioxidants than green olives, and only extra virgin olive oil—the first press of the olives—contains significant amounts of the antioxidants, says Dr. Galli. This is the first solid evidence that eating olives alone, as well as using their oil, can fight disease and slow down aging.

RED WINE VS. HEART DISEASE

Although one widely publicized Harvard study recently suggested that any type of alcoholic beverage in moderation protects against heart disease, the evidence is still most convincing for wine. The main reason: Wine, notably red wine, is the alcoholic beverage with the highest levels of antioxidants. Red wine also exhibits the greatest ability to keep bad LDL cholesterol from being oxidized or able to clog arteries.

The superior antioxidant powers of red wine vs. white wine was recently demonstrated by Edwin Frankel, Ph.D., research chemist at the University of California at Davis. He tested the antioxidant activity of fourteen red and six white California wines. The red wines contained about ten times more antioxidant chemicals, called phenolic compounds, than white wines did. Most important, in Dr. Frankel's test-tube studies, red wine's antioxidants inhibited the dangerous oxidation of bad LDL cholesterol by an astounding 46 percent to 100 percent, compared with only 3 percent to 6 percent for white wine.

Further, a couple of studies suggest that white wine may promote artery damage. Israeli researchers found that drinking white wine spurred a 34 percent jump in dangerous blood fat oxidation and a 41 percent increase in dangerous oxidation of LDL cholesterol in particular. In contrast, red wine depressed blood fat oxidation by 20 percent and LDL oxidation by 40 percent.

Similarly, French studies in animals found that detrimental blood-clotting activity (platelet stickiness or aggregation) was initially depressed by red wine, white wine and straight alcohol. However, fourteen hours later, investigators detected a "rebound effect" from white wine and alcohol. Blood clotting tendency from red wine was still down about 60 percent. But blood stickiness had shot up 46 percent in white wine drinkers and 124 percent in those who drank plain alcohol.

However, one type of white wine, champagne, may be an exception; it appears to have antioxidant, anticlogging benefit, says Dr. Serge Renaud, famed French government researcher. He explains that the antioxidant-containing grape skins are often left in the mix longer when making champagne than when making other white wines.

In a new answer to the question, does drinking alcohol

cause breast cancer, UCLA investigator Matthew P. Long-necker says yes. In a large study of more than sixteen thousand women, he found that women who consumed on average one drink a day over a lifetime upped their risk of breast cancer 39 percent; two drinks a day increased the risk by 69 percent, and about three drinks a day boosted the risk 230 percent. However, there was an exception: Drinking wine in this study did not boost the risk of breast cancer, possibly because of wine's high antioxidant content, researchers said.

Added Iron Danger

There's more evidence that excessive iron may accelerate aging. Neurologists at University Clinic in Innsbruck, Austria, compared the amount of blockage of carotid (neck) arteries in 847 men and women. They found that high stores of iron (ferritin) in tissues was "one of the strongest indicators of carotid artery disease" in both men and women ages forty to seventy. The Austrian researchers also found more extensive carotid artery clogging in men than in women until after age seventy—possibly, they said, because men store more iron than menstruating women.

More Sugar Blues

Excessive sugar could age you prematurely and shorten your life span, according to new animal studies by Roger B. McDonald and colleagues at the University of California at Davis. In a recent series of experiments, they found that rats allowed to eat as much table sugar as they wanted had early deaths. Rats allowed only 60 percent as much table sugar lived about 35 percent longer than rats who freely ate sugar. One explanation might be that the long-lived rats ate many fewer calories; restricting calories is a sure way to prolong survival in animals, but that was not the entire story. Sugar was more lethal, regardless of caloric burden, than starchy carbohydrates. Rats eating an equal number of calories from starch, as found in bread and grains, also outlived excessive sugar-eaters by 20 percent. Researchers theorized that excessive sugar ultimately results in high generation of free radical chemicals that mess up proteins and accelerate the aging process, bringing on disease and premature death. Researchers say the same detrimental biochemical changes suffered by the laboratory animals also happen in humans.

WHERE TO FIND
ANTIAGING SUPPLEMENTS

A Personal Note from the Author

After *Stop Aging Now!* was first published in hardcover in 1995, I was deluged with questions about which types and brand names of antiaging supplements were best, where readers could buy them, and how much they cost. The answers are important, because at the heart of efforts to slow down aging is a specific complement of vitamins, minerals, and other antiaging substances.

Essentially, there are two approaches: You can buy a standard multivitamin-mineral formula, and then add other vitamins, minerals or herbs individually in the higher doses. This can work well for some people. If you are a careful shopper, you can find the right supplements and doses at a reasonable price of around a dollar a day. A drawback for some, however, is taking so many pills a day—at least ten and, ideally, in split doses, as many as fifteen or more.

You can also take a vitamin-mineral formula that combines a variety of nutrients recommended by antiaging experts all in one formula. Several multinutrient products are very good, as far as they go. They may lack certain nutrients, such as coQ-10, or contain lower than ideal doses of other antiaging agents. Also, many are not readily available through traditional consumer outlets or can be quite expensive, running more than three dollars a day or around a hundred dollars a month for a complete formula.

Unfortunately, selecting and taking the supplements can be so confusing, inconvenient, and sometimes costly that some readers said they became discouraged and gave up after a few weeks or a few months.

As a result, a *Stop Aging Now!* multinutrient formula is now in development. It reflects the research findings and recommendations in this book. It is the daily supplement that I myself feel most comfortable taking. It includes everything adults, especially those over age forty, most need in a single overall antiaging supplement. The formula will be changed as necessary, to reflect the latest findings on aging and age-related diseases. The initial cost is not to exceed a dollar a day or thirty dollars for a month's supply.

A portion of the proceeds from the sales of the new formula is also targeted for research on aging; the funds will be donated to the American Aging Association, a leading scientific group on the study of biomedical aspects of aging, and to other appropriate groups in the future.

To get more information about the *Stop Aging Now!* formula that contains the essential antiaging vitamins, minerals, and other substances described in this book, you can call 1-800-627-9721, or write *Stop Aging Now!* Box 311, Waynesboro, PA 17268.

Readers with existing medical conditions (including pregnant women) or who are on medications are encouraged to seek the advice of a qualified medical professional before taking the *Stop Aging Now!* formula. The formula is intended for adults only, not children. The author and publisher expressly disclaim responsibility for any adverse effects resulting from use of the *Stop Aging Now!* formula.

REFERENCES

Much of the material in this book comes from personal inter-views with researchers, papers presented at scientific confer-ences, computer searchs of medical databases of abstracts, medical news reports in both popular and specialized publica-tions, as well as published scientific reports in peer-reviewed journals. It is impossible to note any but a small proportion of the published work on the subject.

Here are some of the important published reports sup-porting the free radical theory of aging and how antioxidants, vitamins and other natural substances can help retard and reverse aging changes.

The articles can be found primarily in medical libraries. Only names of first authors are listed.

AGING, FREE RADICALS AND ANTIOXIDANTS

Agarwal, S. DNA oxidative damage and life expectancy in houseflies. *Proceedings of the National Academy of Sciences* 1994; 91 (25): 12332–35.

Ames, B. N. Oxidants, antioxidants, and the degenerative dis-eases of aging. *Proceedings of the National Academy of Sci-ences* 1993; 90 (17): 7915–22.

Carney, J. M. Aging and oxygen-induced modifications in brain biochemistry and behavior. *Annals of the New York Academy of Sciences* 1994; 738: 44–53.

————. Brain antioxidant activity of spin traps in Mongolian gerbils. *Methods of Enzymology* 1994; 234: 523–26.

Harman, D. Free radical theory of aging: History. In *Free Radicals and Aging,* eds. I. Ement and B. Chance. Basel, Switzerland: Birkhauser Verlag, 1992.

————. The aging process: Major risk factor for disease and death. *Proceedings of the National Academy of Sciences* 1991; 88: 5360–63.

————. Aging: Prospects for further increases in the functional life span. *Age* 1994; 17: 119–46.

Rusting, R. L. Why do we age? *Scientific American* 1992; 267 (6): 130.

Skolnick, A. A. Brain researchers bullish on prospects for preserving mental functioning in elderly. *Journal of the American Medical Association* 1992; 267 (16): 2154.

Smith, C. D. Excess brain protein oxidation and enzyme dysfunction in normal aging and in Alzheimer disease. *Proceedings of the National Academy of Sciences* 1991, December 1; 88 (23): 10540–43.

Walford, R. L. The clinical promise of diet restriction. *Geriatrics* 1990; 45(4): 81–83, 86–87.

Young, S. Against ageing; scientists search for ageing mechanism. *New Scientist* 1993, April 17; 138 (1869): S10.

ALCOHOL AND WINE

Beilin, L. J. Alcohol and hypertension. *Clinical and Experimental Hypertension—Theory and Practice* 1992, A14 (1&2): 119–38.

Criqui, M. H. Does diet or alcohol explain the French paradox? *The Lancet* 1994; 344 (8939–8940): 1719–23.

Doll, R. Mortality in relation to consumption of alcohol: 13 years' observations of male British doctors. *British Medical Journal* 1994; 309 (6959): 911–18.

Frankel, E. N. Inhibition of oxidation of human low density lipoprotein by phenolic substances in red wine. *The Lancet* 1993, February 20; 341: 454–57.

Kinsella, J. E. Possible mechanisms for the protective role of antioxidants in wine and plant foods. *Food Technology* 1993, April: 85–89.

Klatsky, A. L. Epidemiology of coronary heart disease—influence of alcohol. *Alcoholism Clinical and Experimental Research* 1994; 18 (1): 88–97.

Marmot, M. G. Alcohol and blood pressure: the INTERSALT study. *British Medical Journal* 1994; 308 (6939): 1263.

Ridker, P. Association of moderate alcohol consumption and plasma concentration of endogenous tissue-type plasminogen activator. *Journal of the American Medical Association* 1994; 272 (12): 929–33.

Witteman, J. C. Relation of moderate alcohol consumption and risk of systemic hypertension in women. *American Journal of Cardiology* 1990, March 1; 65 (9): 633–37.

Beta Carotene

Comstock, G. W. Serum retinol, beta carotene, vitamin E and selenium as related to subsequent cancer of specific sites. *American Journal of Epidemiology* 1992, January 15; 135 (2): 115–21.

Garewal, H. S. Emerging role of beta-carotene and antioxidant nutrients in prevention of oral cancer. *Archives of Otolaryngology Head Neck Surgery* 1995; 121 (2): 141–44.

Gaziano, J. M. The role of beta-carotene in the prevention of cardiovascular disease. *Annals of the New York Academy of Sciences* 1993, December 31; 691: 148–55.

———. Antioxidant vitamins and coronary artery disease risk. *American Journal of Medicine* 1994, September 26; 97 (3A): 18S–21S.

Hoffman, R. M. Antioxidants and the prevention of coronary heart disease. *Archives of Internal Medicine* 1995, 155 (3): 241–46.

Knekt, P. Serum antioxidant vitamins and risk of cataract. *British Medical Journal* 1992, December 5; 305 (6866): 1392–94.

Manson, J. E. Antioxidants and cardiovascular disease: a review. *Journal of the American College of Nutrition* 1993, August; 12 (4): 426–32.

Mayne, S. T. Dietary beta carotene and lung cancer risk in U.S. nonsmokers. *Journal of the National Cancer Institute* 1994, January 5; 86 (1): 33–38.

Phillips, R. W. B-carotene inhibits rectal mucosal ornithine decarboxylase activity in colon cancer patients. *Cancer Research* 1993; 53: 3723–25.

Prabhala, R. H. Influence of beta-carotene on immune functions. *Annals of the New York Academy of Sciences* 1993, December 31; 691: 262–63.

Prince, M. R. Beta-carotene accumulation in serum and skin. *American Journal of Clinical Nutrition* 1993, February; 57 (2): 175–81.

Schroeder, D. J. Cancer prevention and beta carotene. *The Annals of Pharmacotherapy* 1994, April 28: 470–71.

Street, D. A. Serum antioxidants and myocardial infarction. *Circulation* 1994; 90: 1154–61.

CALCIUM

Barger-Lux, M. J. The role of calcium intake in preventing bone fragility, hypertension and certain cancers. *Journal of Nutrition* 1994; 124: 1406S–11S.

Chapuy, M. C. Vitamin D3 and calcium to prevent hip fractures in elderly women. *New England Journal of Medicine* 1992; 327: 1637–42.

Garland, C. Dietary vitamin D and calcium and risk of colorectal cancer: a 19-year-prospective study in men. *The Lancet* 1985; 2: 307–9.

Hatton, D. C. Dietary calcium and blood pressure in experimental models of hypertension. A review. *Hypertension* 1994, April; 23 (4): 513–30.

McCarron, D. A. Calcium nutrition and hypertensive cardiovascular risk in humans. *Clinical Applied Nutrition* 1992; 2 (4): 45–66.

Sowers, J. R. Calcium metabolism and dietary calcium in salt sensitive hypertension. *American Journal of Hypertension* 1991; 4: 557–63.

Chromium

Abraham, A. S. The effects of chromium supplementation on serum-glucose and lipids in patients with and without non-insulin dependent diabetes. *Metabolism* 1992; 41 (7): 768–71.

Anderson, R. A. Supplemental-chromium effects on glucose, insulin, glucagon and urinary chromium losses in subjects consuming controlled low-chromium diets. *American Journal of Clinical Nutrition* 1991; 54: 909–16.

———. Recent advances in the clinical and biochemical effects of chromium deficiency. *Progress in Clinical and Biological Research* 1993; 380: 221–34.

———. Chromium, glucose tolerance and diabetes. *Biological Trace Element Research* 1992; 32: 19–24.

Evans, G. W. Chromium picolinate increases longevity (abstract). *Age* 1992; 15: 134.

Mertz, W. Chromium in human nutrition: a review. *Journal of Nutrition* 1993; 123: 626–33.

Nestler, J. E. Dehydroepiandrosterone: the missing link between hyperinsulinemia and atherosclerosis? *FASEB Journal* 1992; 6: 3073–75.

Press, R. I. The effect of chromium picolinate on serum cholesterol and apolipoprotein fractions in human subjects. *Western Journal of Medicine* 1990; 152 (1): 41–45.

Reaven, G. M. The role of insulin resistance and hyperinsulinemia in coronary heart disease. *Metabolism* 1992; 41: 16–19.

COENZYME Q-10 (UBIQUINOL)

Baggio, E. Italian multicenter study on the safety and efficacy of coenzyme Q10 as adjunctive therapy in heart failure (interim analysis). *Clinical Investigator* 1993; 71: S145–49.

Coles, L. S. Coenzyme Q-10 and lifespan extension. Paper read at 2nd annual conference on anti-aging medicine and biomedical technology for the year 2010. December 4–6, 1994, Las Vegas, Nevada.

Greenberg, S. Co-enzyme Q10: a new drug for cardiovascular disease. *Journal of Clinical Pharmacology* 1990; 30 (7): 596–608.

Folkers, K. Heart failure is a dominant deficiency of coenzyme A10 and challenges for future clinical research on CoQ10. *Clinical Investigator* 1993; 71 (8 Suppl.): S51–54.

———. Therapy with coenzyme Q10 of patients in heart failure who are eligible or ineligible for a transplant. *Biochemical and Biophysical Research Communications* 1992, January 15; 182 (1): 247–53.

Frei, B. Ubiquinol-10 is an effective lipid-soluble antioxidant at physiological concentrations. *Proceedings of the National Academy of Sciences* 1990; 87: 4879–83.

Lamperitico, M. Italian multicenter study on the efficacy and safety of coenzyme Q10 as adjuvant therapy in heart failure. *Clinical Investigator* 1993; 71: S129–33.

Langsjoen, P. H. Isolated diastolic dysfunction of the myocardium and its response to CoQ-10 treatment. *Clinical Investigator* 1993; 71 (8 Suppl.): S140–42.

Linnane, A. W. Mitochondrial DNA mutation and the ageing process: bioenergy and pharmacological intervention. *Mutation Research* 1992; 275: 195–208.

GARLIC

Amagase, H. Impact of various sources of garlic and their constituents on 7 12-dimethylbenz(a) anthracene binding to mammary cell DNA. *Carcinogenesis* 1993; 14 (8): 1627–31.

Kiesewetter, H. Effects of garlic coated tablets in peripheral arterial occlusive disease. *Clinical Investigator* 1993; 71 (5): 383–86.

Makheja, A. Antiplatelet constituents of garlic and onions. *Agents Actions* 1990; 29 (3–4): 360–63.

McMahon, F. G. Can garlic lower blood pressure? a pilot study. *Pharmacotherapy* 1993; 13 (4): 406–7.

Phelps, S. Garlic supplementation and lipoprotein oxidation susceptibility. *Lipids* 1993, May; 28 (5): 475–77.

Pressing garlic for possible health benefits. *Tufts University Diet and Nutrition Letter*, September 1994; 12 (7): 3.

Silagy, C. Garlic as a lipid lowering agent—a meta-analysis. *Journal of the Royal College of Physicians, London* 1994; 28 (1): 39–45.

Warshafsky, S. Effect of garlic on total serum cholesterol. A meta-analysis. *Annals of Internal Medicine* 1993; 119 (7 Pt. 1): 599–605.

GINKGO BILOBA EXTRACT

Allain, H. Effect of two doses of ginkgo biloba extract (EGb 761) on the dual-coding test in elderly subjects. *Clinical Therapeutics* 1993, May–June; 15 (3): 549–58.

Hoffenberth, B. The efficacy of EGb 761 in patients with senile dementia of the Alzheimer type, a double-blind, placebo-controlled study on different levels of investigation. *Human Psychopharmacology* 1994; 9: 215–22.

Huguet, F. Decreased cerebral 5-HT1A receptors during aging: reversal by Ginkgo biloba extract (EGb761). *Journal of Pharmacy and Pharmacology* 1994; 46: 316–18.

Kleijnen, J. Ginkgo biloba for cerebral insufficiency. *British Journal of Clinical Pharmacology* 1992, October; 34 (4): 352–58.

Oyama, Y. Myricetin and quercetin, the flavonoid constituents of Ginkgo biloba extract, greatly reduce oxidative metabolism in both resting and Ca(2+)-loaded brain neurons. *Brain Research* 1994, January 28; 635 (1–2): 125–29.

Schneider, B. Ginkgo biloba extract in peripheral arterial diseases. Meta analysis of controlled clinical studies. *Arzneimittelforschung* 1992, April; 42 (4): 428–36.

GLUTATHIONE

Aw, T. Y. Intestinal absorption and lymphatic transport of peroxidized lipids in rats: effect of exogenous GSH. *American Journal of Physiology* 1992, November; 263: G665–72.

Julius, M. Glutathione and morbidity in a community-based sample of elderly. *Journal of Clinical Epidemiology* 1994; 47 (9): 1021–26.

Johnston, C. *American Journal of Clinical Nutrition* 1993; 58: 103–5.

Jones, D. P. Glutathione in foods listed in the National Cancer Institute's Health Habits and History Food Frequency Questionnaire. *Nutrition and Cancer* 1992; 17 (1): 57–75.

Kaleric, T. Suppression of human immunodeficiency virus expression in chronically infected monocytic cells by glutathione, glutathione Ester and N-acetylcysteine. *Proceedings of the National Academy of Sciences* 1991, February 1; 88.

Lang, C. A. Glutathione deficiency occurs in 77% of hospital-

, ized subjects of various ages. *Gerontologist* 1990; 30: 39A.

———. Blood glutathione: a biochemical index of life span enhancement in the diet restricted Lobund-Wister rat. In *The Effects of Dietary Restriction on Aging and Disease in the Germ-free and Conventional Lobund-Wister Rat*, ed. D. L. Snyder. New York: Alan R. Liss, 1988.

Meydani, S. N. In vitro glutathione supplementation enhances interleukin-2 production and mitogenic response of peripheral blood mononuclear cells from young and old subjects. *Journal of Nutrition* 1994; 124 (5): 655–63.

Ritchie, J. P. Correction of a glutathione deficiency in the aging mosquito increases its longevity. *Proceedings of the Society for Experimental Biology and Medicine* 1987; 184: 113–17.

Shigenaga, M. K. Oxidative damage and mitochondrial decay in aging. *Proceedings of the National Academy of Sciences* 1994; 91: 10771–78.

MAGNESIUM

Altura, B. Magnesium: growing in clinical importance. *Patient Care* 1994, January 15; 130–50.

Nadler, J. L. Magnesium deficiency produces insulin resistance and increased thromboxane synthesis. *Hypertension* 1993, June; 21 (6, Pt. 2): 1024–29.

Rayssiguier, Y. Magnesium and aging. I. Experimental data: importance of oxidative damage. *Magnesium Research* 1993; 6 (4): 369–78.

Seelig, M. S. Interrelationship of magnesium and estrogen in cardiovascular and bone disorders, eclampsia, migraine and premenstrual syndrome. *Journal of the American College of Nutrition* 1993; 12 (4): 442–58.

Witteman, J. Reduction of blood pressure with oral magnesium supplementation in women with mild to moderate hypertension. *American Journal of Clinical Nutrition* 1994; 50: 129–35.

SELENIUM

Berr, C. Selenium and oxygen-metabolizing enzymes in elderly community residents: a pilot epidemiological study. *Journal of the American Geriatric Society* 1993; 41 (2): 143–48.

Comstock, G. W. Serum retinol, beta carotene, vitamin E and selenium as related to subsequent cancer sites. *American Journal of Epidemiology* 1992; 135 (2): 115–21.

Secor, C. L. Variation in the selenium content of individual Brazil nuts. *Journal of Food Safety* 1989; 9: 279–81.

Tsang, N. C. Serum levels of antioxidants and age-related macular degeneration. *Documenta Ophthalmologica* 1992; 81 (4): 387–400.

van den Brandt, P. A. A prospective cohort study on selenium status and the risk of lung cancer. *Cancer Research* 1993, October 15; 53 (20): 4860–65.

VITAMINS—ANTIOXIDANT AND GENERAL ANTIAGING ACTIVITY

Blot, W. J. Nutrition intervention trials in Linxian, China: supplementation with specific vitamin/mineral combinations, cancer incidence, and disease-specific mortality in the general population. *Journal of the National Cancer Institute* 1993; 85 (18): 1483–92.

Blumberg, J. B. Changing nutrient requirements in older adults. *Nutrition Today* 1992, September; 27 (5): 15.

Buying vitamins: what's worth the price? *Consumer Reports* 1994, September: 565–69.

Hensrud, D. D. Antioxidant status, fatty acids and cardiovascular disease. *Nutrition* 1994, March–April; 10 (2): 170–75.

Lamm, D. L. Megadose vitamins in bladder cancer: a double-blind clinical trial. *Journal of Urology* 1994; 151 (1): 21–26.

Manson, J. E. A prospective study of antioxidant vitamins and incidence of coronary heart disease in women. (Abstract) *Supplement to Circulation* 1992; 84: 4, II 546.

Meyer, F. Lower ischemic heart disease incidence and mortality among vitamin supplement users in a cohort of 2,226 men. 2nd international conference: Antioxidant vitamins and beta-carotene in disease prevention. (Abstract p. 61.) October 10–12, 1994, Berlin.

Riemersma, R. A. Risk of angina pectoris and plasma concentrations of vitamins A, C, and E and carotene. *The Lancet* 1991, January 5; 337 (8732): 1–5.

Russell, R. M. Vitamin requirements of elderly people: an update. *American Journal of Clinical Nutrition* 1993, July; 58 (1): 4–14.

———. Changes in gastrointestinal function attributed to aging. *American Journal of Clinical Nutrition* 1992, June; 55 (6 Suppl.): 1203S–7S.

Seddon, J. M. The use of vitamin supplements and the risk of cataract among US male physicians. *American Journal of Public Health* 1994; 84: 788–92.

Sperduto, R. D. The Linxian cataract studies. *Archives of Ophthalmology* 1993; 111: 1246–53.

VITAMIN B: FOLIC ACID, B6, B12

Healton, E. B. Neurological aspects of cobalamin deficiency. *Medicine* (Baltimore) 1991, July; 70 (4): 229–45.

Heimburger, D. C. Localized deficiencies of folic acid in aerodigestive tissues. *Annals of the New York Academy of Sciences* 1992, September 30; 669: 87–95.

Heseker, H. Psychological disorders as early symptoms of a mild-to-moderate vitamin deficiency. *Annals of the New York Academy of Sciences* 1992, September 30; 669: 352–57.

Meydani, S. N. Vitamin B-6 and immune competence. *Nutrition Review* 1993; 51 (8): 217–25.

Selhub, J. Vitamin status and intake as primary determinants of homocysteinemia in an elderly population. *Journal of the American Medical Association* 1993; 270: 2693–98.

Stampfer, M. J. Homocysteine and marginal vitamin deficiency: the importance of adequate vitamin intake: Editorial. *Journal of the American Medical Association* 1993; 270 (22): 2726.

Vitamin C

Block, G. Vitamin C and cancer prevention: the epidemiologic evidence. *American Journal of Clinical Nutrition* 1991; 53: 270S–82S.

Cheraskin, E. Vitamin C: who needs it? *Journal of Naturopathic Medicine* 1993; 4 (1): 81–83.

Enstrom, J. E. Vitamin C intake and mortality among a sample of the United States population. *Epidemiology* 1992; 3: 194–202.

———. Vitamin C intake and mortality among a sample of the United States population: new results. In *Biological Oxidants and Antioxidants*, ed. Lester Packer. Stuttgart: Hippokrates Verlag, 1994.

Feldman, E. B. Ascorbic acid supplements and blood pressure—a four week pilot study. *Annals of the New York Academy of Sciences* 1992; 669: 342–48.

Frei, B. Ascorbate is an outstanding antioxidant in human blood plasma. *Proceedings of the National Academy of Sciences* 1989; 86: 6377–81.

Jacques, P. Effects of vitamin C on high density lipoprotein cholesterol and blood pressure. *Journal of the American College of Nutrition* 1992; 62: 252–55.

King, G. Rate of excretion of vitamin C in human urine. *Age* 1994; 17: 1–6.

Newton, H. M. The cause and correction of low blood vitamin C concentrations in the elderly. *American Journal of Clinical Nutrition* 1985; 42 (4): 656–69.

VITAMIN E

Gey, K. F. Inverse correlation between plasma vitamin E and mortality from ischemic heart disease in cross-cultural epidemiology. *American Journal of Clinical Nutrition* (suppl.) 1991; 53: 326S–34S.

Jialal, I. The effect of dietary supplementation with alpha-tocopherol on the oxidative modification of low density lipoprotein. *Journal of Lipid Research* 1992; 6: 899–906.

———. The effect of a-tocopherol supplementation on LDL oxidation and vitamin E: a dose response study. *Arteriosclerosis, Thrombosis and Vascular Biology* 1995: 15 (2): 190–98.

Mayne, S. T. Dietary beta carotene and lung cancer risk in U.S. nonsmokers. *Journal of the National Cancer Institute* 1994; 86 (1): 33–38.

Meydani, M. Vitamin E. Health benefits. *The Lancet* 1995, January 21; 345 (8943): 170–76.

Rimm, E. B. Vitamin E consumption and the risk of coronary heart disease in men. *New England Journal of Medicine* 1993; 328: 1450–56.

Stampfer, M. J. Vitamin E consumption and the risk of coronary disease in women. *New England Journal of Medicine* 1993; 328: 1444–49.

FISH, MEAT AND FATS

Burr, M. K. L. Effects of changes in fat, fish and fibre intakes on death and myocardial reinfarctions: diet and reinfarction trial (DART). *The Lancet* 1989; 2: 757–61.

Kromhout, D. The inverse relation between fish consumption and 20-year mortality from coronary heart disease. *New England Journal of Medicine* 1985; 312: 1205–9.

Lands, W. E. Biochemistry and physiology of n-3 fatty acids. *FASEB Journal* 1992; 6: 2530–36.

Sugimura, T. Heterocyclic amines in cooked foods: candidates for causation of common cancers. *Journal of the National Cancer Institute* 1994; 86 (1): 2–4.

Wang Y. Y. Formation of mutagens in cooked foods. V. The mutagen reducing effect of soy protein concentrates and antioxidants during frying of beef. *Cancer Letters* 1982; 16: 179–89.

Weisburger, J. H. Prevention of heterocyclic amine formation in relation to carcinogenesis. In *Mutagens in Food: Detection and Prevention*, ed. H. Hayatsu. Boca Raton, Fla.: CRC Press, 1991.

Willett, W. C. Relation of meat, fat and fiber intake to the risk of colon cancer in a prospective study among women. *New England Journal of Medicine* 1990; 323: 1664–72.

———. Intake of trans fatty acids and risk of coronary heart disease among women. *The Lancet* 1993; 341: 581–85.

IRON

Nelson, R. L. Body iron stores and risk of colonic neoplasia. *Journal of the National Cancer Institute* 1994; 86 (6): 455–60.

Salonen, J. T. High stored iron levels are associated with excess risk of myocardial infarction in eastern Finnish men. *Circulation* 1992; 86: 803–11.

ZINC

Boukaiba, N. A physiological amount of zinc supplementation: effects on nutritional, lipid, and thymic status in an elderly population. *American Journal of Clinical Nutrition* 1993; 57: 566–72.

Chandra, R. K. Excessive intake of zinc impairs immune responses. *Journal of the American Medical Association* 1984; 252: 1443–46.

Fabris, N. Biomarkers of aging in the neuroendocrine-immune domain. Time for a new theory of aging? *Annals of the New York Academy of Sciences* 1992; 663: 335–48.

Grasso, G. Restorative effect of thymomodulin and zinc on interferon-gamma production in aged mice. *Annals of the New York Academy of Sciences* 1992; 673: 256–59.

Kaminski, M. S. Evaluation of dietary antioxidant levels and supplementation with two commercial formulas. *Journal of the American Optometric Association* 1993; 64 (12): 862–70.

Prasad, A. S. Zinc deficiency in elderly patients. *Nutrition* 1993; 9: 218–24.

FRUITS AND VEGETABLES

Block, G. Fruit, vegetables and cancer prevention: A review of the epidemiologic evidence. *Nutrition and Cancer* 1992; 18: 1–29.

———. The data support a role for antioxidants in reducing cancer risk. *Nutrition Reviews* 1992; 50: 207–13.

Giovannucci, E. F. methionine and alcohol intake and risk of colorectal adenoma. *Journal of the National Cancer Institute* 1993; 85: 875–84.

Glynn, S. A. Folate and cancer: A review of the literature. *Nutrition and Cancer* 1994; 22: 101–19.

Patterson, B. H. Fruit and vegetables in the American Diet: data from the NHANES II survey. *American Journal of Public Health* 1990; 80: 1443–49.

Steinmetz, K. A. Vegetables, fruit, and cancer, part I: epidemiology. *Cancer Causes Control* 1991; 2: 325–27.

———. Vegetables, fruit and cancer, part II: mechanisms. *Cancer Causes Control* 1991; 2: 427–42.

Supplement to *The American Journal of Clinical Nutrition.* Proceedings of the second international congress on vegetarian nutrition. May 1994; 59 (5S): 1099S–1262S.

Vegetarianism—Live longer. *British Medical Journal* 1994; 308: 1667–771.

White, R. Health effects and prevalence of vegetarianism. *Western Journal of Medicine* 1994; 160 (5): 465.

SOYBEANS

Barnes, S. Soybeans inhibit mammary tumor growth in models of breast cancer. In *Mutagens and Carcinogens in the Diet,* ed. M. W. Pariza, New York: Wiley-Liss, 1990.

Carroll K. K. Review of clinical studies on cholesterol-lowering response to soy protein. *Journal of the American Dietetics Association* 1991; 91: 820–27.

Messina, M. The role of soy products in reducing risk of cancer. *Journal of the National Cancer Institute* 1991; 83: 541–46.

Santiago, L. A. Japanese soybean paste miso scavenges free radicals and inhibits lipid peroxidation. *Journal of Nutritional Science and Vitaminology* 1992; 38: 297–304.

Sirtori, C.R. Soybean protein diet and plasma cholesterol: from therapy to molecular mechanisms. *Annals of the New York Academy of Sciences* 1993; 676: 188–201.

Troll, W. Soybean diet lowers breast tumor incidence in irradiated rats. *Carcinogenesis* 1980; 1: 469–72.

You, W. C. Diet and high risk of stomach cancer in Shandong, China. *Cancer Research* 1988; 48: 3518–23.

TEA

Gao, Y. T. Reduced risk of esophageal cancer associated with green tea consumption. *Journal of the National Cancer Institute* 1994; 86 (11): 855–58.

Hertog, M. Dietary antioxidant flavonoids and risk of coronary heart disease: the Zutphen elderly study. *The Lancet* 1993; 342: 1007–11.

Sato, Y. Possible contribution of green tea drinking habits to the prevention of stroke. *Tohoku Journal of Experimental Medicine* 1989; 157 (4): 337–43.

Serafini, M. Red wine, tea and antioxidants. *The Lancet* 1994; 344: 626.

Shibata, A. A prospective study of pancreatic cancer in the elderly. *International Journal of Cancer* 1994, July 1; 58 (1): 46–49.

Sohn, O. S. Effects of green and black tea on hepatic xenobiotic metabolizing systems in the male F344 rat. *Xenobiotica* 1994; 24 (2): 119–27.

Yang, C. S. Tea and cancer. *Journal of the National Cancer Institute* 1993; 85 (13): 1038–49.

Books

Bliznakov, Emile G., M.D., and Hunt, Gerald L. *The Miracle Nutrient Coenzyme Q10.* New York: Bantam Books, 1986.

Canfield, Louise M. *Carotenoids in Human Health.* New York: Annals of the New York Academy of Sciences, Volume 691, 1993.

Carper, Jean. *Food—Your Miracle Medicine.* New York: Harper-Collins, 1993.

———. *The Food Pharmacy.* New York: Bantam Books, 1988.

Cheraskin, Emanuel, M.D. *Vitamin C: Who Needs It?* Birmingham, Ala.: Arlington Press & Company, 1993.

Garland, Cedric, and Garland, Frank, with Ellen Thro. *The Calcium Connection.* New York: Fireside, 1989.

Hayflick, Leonard. *How and Why We Age.* New York: Ballantine Books, 1994.

Hausman, Patricia, M.S. *The Right Dose.* Emmaus, Penn.: Rodale Press, 1987.

Littarru, Gian Paolo. *Energy and Defense: Facts and Perspectives on Coenzyme Q10 in Biology and Medicine.* Rome, Italy: Casa Editrice Scientifica Internazionale, 1994.

Messina, Mark, Ph.D.; Messina, Virginia, R.D.; Setchell, Kenneth, D.R., Ph.D. *The Simple Soybean and Your Health.* Garden City, N.Y.: Avery Publishing Group, 1994.

Shabert, Judy, M.D., R.N., and Ehrlich, Nancy. *The Ultimate Nutrient Glutamine: The Essential Nonessential Amino Acid.* Garden City Park, N.Y.: Avery Publishing Group, 1994.

Tyler, Varro E., Ph.D. *Herbs of Choice.* Binghamton, N.Y.: Pharmaceutical Products Press, 1994.

Walford, Roy L. *The 120-Year Diet.* New York: Pocket Books, 1986.

INDEX

Abrams, Steven A., 101
ACE inhibitors, 162
Acorn squash, 132
Addiction to alcohol, 231
Adler, William, 92, 93
Adlercreutz, Herman, 194
Aging, 1–2, 251–52
    prevention instead of treatment,
      6–7
    references on, 319–20, 328–29
    research and theories on, 2–7,
      9–22, 24, 26, 33–35. *See also*
      Free radical theory
      geriatric gerbil experiment,
      20–22
    vitamin supplement strategy,
      305–10
    when to start, 313
AIDS
    glutathione and, 127
    selenium and, 117, 120–21, 307
Ajoene, 161
Albacore. *See* Tuna
Albumin, 95–96
Alcohol, 226–35, 312. *See also* Beer;
    Wine
    addiction to, 231
    blood pressure and, 296
    brain damage and, 230–31
    cancer and, 229–30, 291
    facts about, 227
    heart disease and, 228
    insulin and, 285
    mental functions and, 228–29
    in moderation, 226–27, 229,
      234–35, 263
    references on, 320–21
    strokes and, 228

Alliance for Aging Research, 45,
    54–55, 61
Allicin, 163, 164–65
Almonds, 114, 116, 214, 262
Alpha tocopherol, 47. *See also* Vit-
    amin E
Alzheimer's disease, 254–55
    coenzyme Q-10 and, 144
    ginkgo and, 153
    vitamin B12 and, 5, 70–71
    vitamin E and, 45, 254–56
American Association of Retired
    Persons' (AARP) 101 Hi-
    Potency supplement, 316–17
Ames, Bruce N., 3, 14, 16, 38, 140,
    141, 168, 251
    vitamins and daily dosages taken
      by, 134
Amino acids, 24, 36. *See also*
    Homocysteine
    glutathione and, 124, 126, 129
    soybeans and, 190, 195
    supplements. *See* Glutamine; L-
      carnitine
Amyotrophic lateral sclerosis
    (ALS). *See* Lou Gehrig's dis-
    ease
Anchovies, 186
Anderson, Richard A., 84–86,
    284–85
Angina (chest pain), 34, 114, 310.
    See also Heart disease
Angiogenesis, 190
Angioplasty, 183
Antacids, 77
Anthocyanins, 175
Antiaging hormone, DHEA (dehy-
    droepiandrosterone), 88